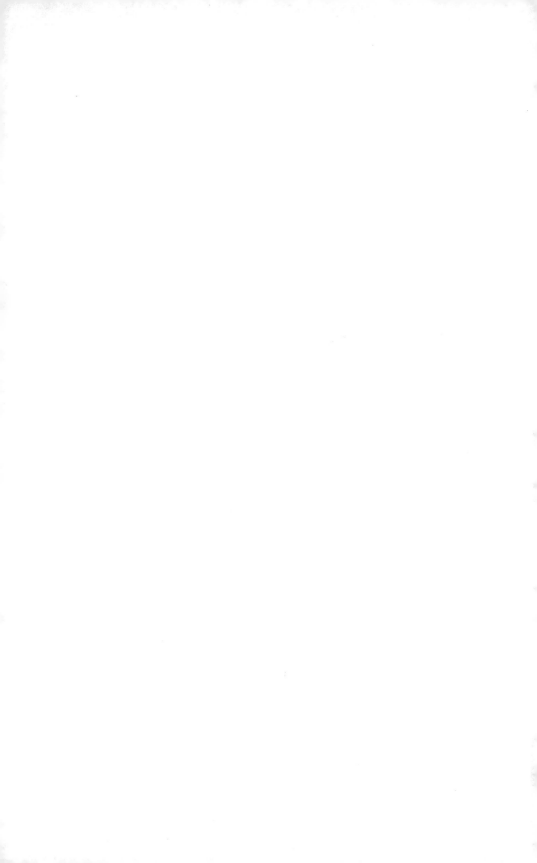

Nekkid

Frank M. Lee

Cincinnati Book Publishing

Nekkid

Frank M. Lee

Connie Breitbeil, coeditor
Connie Lee, coeditor

First Edition, 2013
Copyright © 2013 by Constance Breitbeil

———

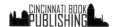
Cincinnati Book Publishing
Anthony W. Brunsman, President
Cincinnati, OH 45202
www.cincybooks.com

Publication

Karen Bullock, project manager
Anthony Brunsman, production and marketing
Brent Beck, cover design

Photographs

Front cover photo from iStock
Front jacket flap from The Paris Post-Intelligencer
Insert photographs from Cleveland Magazine, The Lansing State Journal,
The Paris Post-Intelligencer, and The National Polio Society Newsletter

———

Cataloging and ordering

Library of Congress Control Number: 2013951665
Library of Congress Cataloging-in-Publication Data

Lee, Frank M., 1943 – 2012
Nekkid

ISBN 978-0-9910077-0-7 hardcover

1. American literature—memoir. 2. American literature—Regional—Tennessee. 3. American
Literature—Treatment of Special Subjects—Polio. I. Title.

For additional copies of this book, please contact conniebreitbeil@yahoo.com

Preface

I don't know what the truth is about anything; all I know is what I remember. And my memories are the stuff from which fantastic – in the literal sense – stories are woven, which explains why I've taken up weaving, I suppose.

What you see here, dear reader, is a digest of the stories I've imagined I lived through these years of my life. I cannot vouch for the veracity of any of these stories, therefore out of necessity, I must tell you here are some good yarns which I think you'll enjoy, but they're not based on fact. They're based on my wild and crazy fancy, figments of my imagination.

I thought I was launching genuine memories of a wasted life, but a couple of memory misadventures - my own memory - pointed the way to the fiction section of the library to me. Dramatically.

My older brother Jacky died in nineteen-ninety-six. During my last visit to see him I took a drive through memory lanes we'd paved. I repeatedly tried, without any success, to discuss some of my most cherished memories I had of times spent with him.

"Remember our dog Snowball and how dad dropped her off in a park on our way to Michigan in that old

Desoto? With you and me lying on top of the backseat filled with clothes?"

"No, I don't remember that or anything like it."

"Remember how dad and Annie Catherine used to argue all the time and how you and I would talk about who we'd rather go with if they split up? And you always said you'd go with dad and I said I wanted to go with Annie Catherine?"

"No, Frankie. I don't remember that."

"Remember the day we ran away from the log house out there by Whitlock? How the door to the house was locked when we got home and nobody was there and how we held hands and walked down the road to the neighbors and how they fed us cornbread and something and then drove us into Puryear to the Washatorium where Aunt Louise and Uncle Nolan came and took us to grandmother's?"

"I think you've got a wild imagination, boy. That's what I think. Nothing like that ever happened to me." I shut up.

In nineteen-ninety-nine I told a friend I'd found a book she'd love, "The Farm She Was". "What a coincidence," she grinned. "That's one of my favorite books in the world."

"What am I going to do with the copy I ordered for you, then?"

"It won't be wasted. Pass it around or give it to me and I'll pass it around."

A week later Elaine called. "You've got my book. I've been looking all over for it since we last talked. I distinctly remember I gave it to you."

"No you didn't. I saw it advertised in a catalog, thought you'd like it and have been holding it for you."

"Check out the copy you've got there. I bet you'll see there are comments written in it by me."

"Okay, but I'm absolutely sure."

I telephoned her. "It's your book. You're right. I'm wrong. I've never been so positive about something of which there has not been a scintilla of truth."

These are the fancies of a fanciful old man.

-- Flee

DEDICATION...

This book is dedicated to all the Connies in Frank's life. The first one, his father, whose presence and absence helped shape him into the man he grew to be. The second one, his daughter, who learned from him that love IS more important that all the other stuff. The third one, his partner who loved him, and allowed him to find his happiness.

For you: Kid, Dad, Flee... we miss you.

Born, Frankie Lee Moody
4.13.1943

~

Died, Frank Moody Lee
9.21.2012

Hard to Say

Somebody leaning over the kid. Changing his diaper. Dark hair. Smiling. Cooing. A familiar face handling his butt with familiar hands in a familiar routine. Wait. Wait. Not just yet. Off comes the dirty diaper. Wait.

Strong fingers wrap themselves around his ankles and pull his butt up from the bed. Now! Now! Got her! Right in the face. It's dripping. She's giggling as she scolds him. She thinks he didn't know what he was doing. She'd be wrong.

Sitting on a steep hill in front of a house. The Kid runs up and down and down up and down until something happens to the big toe on his right foot. Blood is spewing. Jacky crying. The Kid spies the culprit. A razor blade lying in the grass. Bloodied.

The Kid sitting in a dining room, his knees pulled up to his chin. Leaning against the wall. He sees his own footprints in the fresh wax on the floor and grins.

His mother has told him to stay away from the wax until it dries. He calls her. "Momma!" "Momma!" She comes, a frown furrowing across her brow, knowing in her heart what's going to happen. "I done did it. Momma, I done did it." Her left arm, hard-muscled from much practice, grabs the Kid by the right arm, raises him into the air and dangles him while the right hand smacks his left buttocks until his left buttocks is bright red. Both know it won't be the last time.

A Headlong Drive

"I'm gonna get me a chopping ax and chop his head off and feed it to the hogs." He talked tough. Hell, the Kid was tough. He'd done all his growing on a farm, butting heads with billy goats and his brother Jacky. He was three years old and he knew what he wanted and what he'd have to do to get it.

What he wasn't going to get, if he could help it, was another baby. Nossir, he wasn't about to give up his role as baby-of-the-family-who-got-the-pampering without a fight.

Three years old and feisty as he'd ever be, the Kid wasn't taking the birth of his latest sibling sitting down. Or the way they'd shunt him aside and ignore him in all the hoopla. Over what? A baby? Now they're doing it. Spoiling his whole life for him. You know mom wasn't going to have any more time for him. Everybody pays their attention to the baby after they've taken it away from the rest of the kids.

They took him over to the Watsons who owned the next farm over. Until Ronald Henry popped out to make his acquaintance known to Henry County, Tennessee. Mr. Alva, who just about everybody called "Alvie", was his keeper and would be for the years they'd know each other.

It was Mr. Watson who gave the Kid his first chaw of tobacco at age five or six and made him sick as a dog and laughed at him while he puked. They were buddies.

Mr. Watson just laughed at the Kid's threat. "Now anytime you get tired of that new baby you just come over here and we'll see what we can do about it. You hear me, boy?"

They were sitting outside the big shed located between the house and the barn where Mr. Watson and his son Lomas kept all their tools. Later it would be a treasure trove of delights for the Kid whenever he came to visit, opening up to exploration for rusty nails, broken hammers, handleless hoes and so much other stuff you couldn't imagine the delights of until you had pillaged that shed at least once. Unpainted weathered siding topped by sheets of rusting corrugated tin. A heavy wooden door that creaked just like a dungeon door and slammed like it never intended to let you out of prison. Ever again.

A neat place.

The Watson's farm was located on a side road out in the country between Paris and Puryear. It looped around from U.S. 641 up by Pete Valentine's place through a couple dozen farms and back onto U.S. 641.

The house was built on a big hill that rose from the creek that ran alongside the gravel road in the front. The creek where the Kid once saw Lomas shoot a water moccasin clear through the head and clear through a frog the water moccasin was swallowing at the time.

A dirt road ran around the base of the hill to the barn. Just the other side of that little road was a cold water spring where the Watsons got their drinking water and where they kept their milk cool so it wouldn't spoil until the milkman could pick it up.

Every day Mr. Watson and Lomas put whatever milk they could in a five gallon stainless steel milk can. A couple of times a week the milkman, in his big refriger-ated truck, would come by and pick up the full can of milk and leave an empty which he'd picked up last trip.

That milk gave the Watsons and thousands of other small farmers some of the cash they desperately needed to exist from harvest to harvest.

And ice. There wasn't any electricity and no re-frigerators, but iceboxes were just about as good. That big brown insulated cabinet on the back porch where they kept butter and the other stuff that would have spoiled had it not been kept cool. And it smelled like a fishy smell would smell if it didn't smell fishy but still smelled.

There was a special cubbyhole for the ice which took the heat off the food. And since one block of ice, say one-and-a-half feet by ten inches, wouldn't last more than three or four days in the hundred degree tempera-tures of July and August, and since replacing it was not free because there weren't enough hard freezes to chop your own ice in the wintertime and preserve it for sum-mertime, the Watsons and just about everybody else the Kid would know during those early years bought ice. More than probably with some of their milk money.

The iceman drove a truck, a big flatbed with side-boards on it. The ice was covered with a big tarpaulin. One of the Kid's delights was running down to meet the iceman with a nickel for a soda. Rena Mae, Mr. Alvie's daughter, just about always made sure he had that nickel.

And he ran down that hill full tilt often going so fast he tumbled all over himself, ass-over-teakettle, in his haste to behold the treasures of the iceman. There were cold drinks, and candy and chewing gum. Hell, a kid could hide under that tarpaulin and, if he didn't freeze to death, live forever on the delicacies carefully concealed thereunder.

Rena Mae was one of the Kid's very favorites. He loved that woman. She really spoiled him. Whenever he was there overnight he slept with Rena Mae. He followed Rena Mae wherever she went. All the rest would shoo him away when he bugged them too much. Not Rena Mae. "Okay, sugar, come on."

Miss Clyde was Mr. Watson's wife.

Miss Clyde slept next to her canary.

Miss Clyde did not sleep next to Mr. Watson.

Miss Clyde did not sleep in the same room with Mr. Watson.

She had a daybed in the living room in the far corner. A tiny bed next to the bird cage and out of the way of the little table that held the battery-powered radio. Not a transistor job. Nossir, this was a far cry from those modern day fancy jobbers. It was a big old wooden radio, a foot high, connected to an antenna wire which ran up a ten foot tobacco stick outside the side window and powered by a battery that must have weighed five pounds.

The batteries were expensive; the Watsons didn't use that radio a whole lot except for farm news and country music. Money wasn't something folks threw around like hickory nuts because there wasn't all that much milk in Henry County. So they were thrifty. And saved some battery power for tomorrow. And next week.

The living room was heated by a fireplace which is also where Rena Mae used to heat up her iron to iron clothes. Even in the summer you'd have to build a fire and set the heavy iron iron on its lower edge, tilted back

5

on the handle so the flames would heat the bottom. In the days before wash and wear.

And popped popcorn and roasted regular corn at night. To eat as family members swapped stories of the day and their lives. In the firelight and in the glow of kerosene lamps. Coal oil. That's what they called kerosene. And every night someone would have to trim the wicks and clean the chimneys which built up lots of lamp black.

Rena Mae's room was the other room. It had a nice bed in it and was the coziest room in the house, filled with essence of Rena Mae, a magic elixir which made the Kid happy. Rena Mae most of the time wouldn't even make him wash his feet before he stuck them under her clean covers.

Later he would feel a whole lot of shame and guilt for not having visited Rena Mae when she was dying.

Lomas and Mr. Watson slept in separate beds in the back bedroom. Both beds had featherbeds you could bury yourself in. After the Kid got older, he was guided by Rena Mae — probably righteously mindful of his precocious prepubescent libido — to share Mr. Watson's bed, which was also delightful. No worry. No matter how cold it got that featherbed kept him toasty warm.

The kitchen was the fourth room, though not the least of them. A big table always filled with homemade jelly and butter and other goodies that a kid would kick shins to get at. Wooden cabinets. None built in. Holding dishes and pots and pans and bottles and glasses and just about anything else anyone could possibly want.

The magic kitchen with its milk gravy on biscuits in the morning, with its sugar on buttered biscuits in mid-morning and Miss Clyde's stewed potatoes at dinner and supper. Cooked on a wood cookstove. Miss Clyde and Rena Mae could cook and the Kid always was up for a meal, particularly supper which was eaten after dark when Lomas and Mr. Watson had come in from the fields after their evening chores of milking and feeding in the barn.

The table was set and flickering in the yellow glow of the coal oil lamps. And no matter what the main course was the Kid would most and longest remember the smell of those stewed potatoes and how they tasted with that wonderful cornbread.

The day's cooking was done in the morning so that the kitchen, and the house, would be cool at night. That's why some folks who had money and time used to build "summer" kitchens, little buildings away from the main house so they could cook without lighting a furnace in the living area.

So here the Kid is, awaiting the birth of his sibling in the red brick-siding house he shares with sister Peggy, brother Jacky, dad Connie and mom Ruby Gordon. And he's thinking he's really pissed because now there's gonna be another brother or sister something or the other. I mean he's got plenty of company already. There's a milk goat that he and Jacky play with and a billy goat that they butt heads with. Why do they need a baby? Maybe mom made a mistake.

"I'll just stay with you, Mr. Watson. I don't want to go home to no new baby. I don't want no baby boy. I don't want no baby girl. I'll just stay here. With you."

His eyes pleading.

But no. Mr. Watson takes his hand and leads the Kid down to the barn where he's repairing harness for

7

the mules. As Mr. Watson picks up the great collar and leans back against the wall of a stall he glances down at the Kid. "You know, boy, there is one thing here that you haven't figured out. If they bring a baby over to your house you're going to have somebody you can boss, just like Peggy Joyce and Jacky boss you. You'll have somebody littler than you that you can tell what to do and what not to do."

"Have you thought about that? Don't you want to be a boss too?"

"There's nobody else little enough for you to boss right now, because you're the littlest there is. The billy goat pushes you around. Even the nanny goat pushes you around."

"If I wuz you, I'd think about that."

The Kid went tearing out of there to tell Rena Mae.

"I'm gonna have somebody to boss, Rena Mae. I'm gonna have somebody to boss when they bring that baby to my house."

"I thought you was gonna chop its head off, sugar, and feed it to the pigs. You'd rather have somebody to play with I see."

"Yep."

It was wash day and Rena Mae was up to her eyes. First she had to build a fire in the fire pit dug for that purpose, then hang a big kettle, filled with water, by a pole hooked onto forked sticks over the fire. Then she'd boil the clothes after shaving homemade lye soap liberally over them, stirring them all the while with a long stick that had been cut for that purpose. After the boil, the clothes had to be rinsed in cold water and hung out on the line to dry.

White clothes had an extra step. In addition to the lye soap she tossed into the boiling water a tightly closed tobacco sack which contained small balls of something blue called blueing. This blueing mixed with grey dirt and unwhiteness to create shiny whiteness, so the theory went. And the theory still goes.

Look inside the boxes holding undepleted supplies of some the popular detergents today and see the blue crystals of blueing just like the stuff Rena Mae used to use. It's been around a long time.

The wash kettle, which must have held a good ten gallons or more, was a multi-purpose utilitarian utensil. After hog killings it was used to render the fat for soap and for making other byproducts from the hog, as well as heating the water to dip the hogs in to get the hair off the body. Lye soap is made from lye and hog fat, and, perhaps, something else which the Kid didn't know about.

Two days later Rena Mae and Mr. Watson walked the Kid down the hill and up the road home. His heart was in his mouth as Rena Mae pushed him inside the door to the front room where his mom was sitting up in bed. But where's the baby?

"Come here to mommy, Kid." She embraced him, hugging him so hard he could hardly breathe. "I missed you," she said. "You're my little man. Now look at what I brought for you."

She turned to her left, picked up a long bundle wrapped in white and gently brought it around to the Kid. "This is your baby brother, Kid. Here's somebody you can play with and have fun with, somebody you can love just like Jacky and Peggy love you. Go on. Hug him. His name is Ronald. Look at him. He loves you already, Kid. Isn't he so sweet?"

The Kid felt the bile of disappointment rising in his throat. He was being shoved aside for the baby and he knew it. Things can never be the way they were. Mom has somebody else she likes as much as she likes me. Nothing will ever be the same again. He was right. They weren't.

Years later he knew he had been right.

Fifty years later when he loved that baby damn nearly as much as his mom had on that October morning in nineteen-forty-six.

Ding Dong the Mom is Dead

The Kid was confused. He was in a strange building with swinging doors.

Dad was howling like he was going crazy. Peggy and Ronald had been taken away. Mom wasn't here to tell him what was happening, and even his imaginative brain hadn't figured out how an exciting trip to town had exploded into a nightmare in a hospital in Paris.

Just an hour ago his mom had stood his irrepressible three year old body on the bed and dressed him up in those pink overall shorts to go to town. His mom with her Sutton-dark hair framing a moon face that looked so much sterner than it was, even when he was a rascal, which he was a lot.

She combed his hair, picked him up under his arms and stood him on the floor by the front door. "Now behave, Kid, until the rest of us are ready to go. If I see one speck of dirt on those britches I'll spank you. I mean it, Kid. I'll just be a few minutes." And off she went to see that Jacky and Peggy were presentable. Jacky was five and Peggy eight. And baby Ronald who, even though he was six months old, still hadn't got the hang of dressing up for a Saturday night in downtown Puryear, Tennessee, so most of the time mom had to do it for him.

The Kid was ready to go. His face felt like the skin had been rubbed raw in the interest of cleanliness. His clothes were stiff from starch and the fresh touch of an iron. What else he felt was about five pounds lighter from the loss of all the grime and dirt mom had scrubbed off him. He was so light he could jump over the barn. He could jump over the woodpile out back.

Why not? The Kid exploded through the screen door onto the front porch. *We're going to town! We're going to town!* The music reverberated through his skull, slithering down his legs where it translated itself into an Irish jig sending him leaping into the front yard, ignoring the three steps between it and him.

We're going to town! We're going to town! He skittered through the yard as night quickly fell on the Hancock place where the family had moved right after Ronald was born.

He loved it here. Everything was so much bigger than it was over at the red brick-siding house. The back porch was screened in. The front porch ran all the way across the front of the house, just like at the Watsons. The yard was as big as a sweet potato field except it had cedar trees instead of potato plants.

The Kid would never run out of places to explore and play here. There was even a pear tree out by the garden and he'd see to it that not a lot of them ever made their way into the house. Nossir, as long as he needed ammunition to ward off attacking Indians, all too many of whom seemed to favor his brother Jacky a lot, and as long as he had an empty gut that needed stuffing five or six times a day — mom would be lucky to save any of those pears for drying or for preserves.

As he ran around the house like a little demon casting a serious spell of mischief, the Kid spotted the big tree roots he'd been playing in earlier that day. His mom's threats forgotten, he bounded over to dig up some more of that red clay dirt for the fort he was making. About the same time Jacky came out of the house with that scrubbed going-to-town look, eyes and hair shining like they had just been waxed. The Kid motioned Jacky over. Making a fort was a two man job. Now they could really get some work done.

"Kid!"

"Kid!"

"Kid, you better get yourself here right this minute and you'd better be clean and have clean clothes on."

"Right now."

"You come here, too, Jacky." Jacky was a lot better at minding than the Kid would ever be. When someone told the Kid to do something he'd say or act "no" and then they'd have to come out to wherever he was making mischief and drag him into the house. Not Jacky. By the time he was five he was pretty well socialized, especially when it came to eating.

The Kid's body jerked as his mind skidded back to another reality and ran just as happily toward the old pick-up truck parked by the big chimney on the east side of the house.

Everybody else was already waiting for the two boys. Dad was behind the wheel. Peggy was standing between mom and dad. Mom was holding Ronald like some precious trinket she was afraid might break. There wasn't room for everybody to sit down in the little cab of the pickup, so the Kid stood. He was the shortest, next to Ronald and you know nobody was gonna make Ronald stand. Jacky next to the Kid.

And off they went, leaving a rooster-tail of dust in their darkening wake as they passed Pete Valentine's house at the bottom of the hill and around the curve and wound their way to highway U.S. 641 a half mile down the road.

13

The Kid got a little scared every time he passed Pete Valentine's house, for he knew that every Saturday night Pete would line up all half dozen of his kids and his wife Bernice and lay into them with a big willow switch. Beat 'em. For all of their sins of the past week. The Kid just knew if he got too close Pete Valentine would grab him and throw him in line, too.

At the highway, dad brought the truck to a full stop, brakes carefully applied to avoid unnecessary bruises and abrasions, looked both ways, then turned right.

Only four miles to Puryear. Population somewhere under three hundred. As small towns go, Puryear, Tennessee was big enough to be one.

Still, in the forties it was a warm, inviting place beckoning area farm families on a Saturday night for basic shopping and fellowship. Everybody'd have a good time. Adults and kids alike. And they knew it. Grocery shopping was an exciting experience for the kids who didn't get to town more than once or twice a month.

Then they'd be sitting around at Rhodies while the adults gossiped. About the weather and the crops and people who'd done something worth talking about. And maybe a cold drink for the kids. Rhodie had a neat Coca Cola cooler right by where she sat and when you paid her your nickel she'd open up the lid and let you fish your own bottle out. Rhodies was self-serve. You got what you wanted and brought it over to Rhodie who would add it up and either put it on your bill or take your bills in payment. And never miss a beat in a conversation with the folks sitting around while she did it.

Although Rhodies was thrilling to the kids, if they'd been older and more cynical they would have seen

14

the store was rundown. The scent of Rhodies was unmistakable. Kinda musty. Kinda mustardy. Kinda sweet. All Rhodies.

The Kid wasn't sure what the walls looked like bare 'cause they were covered from coast to coast with everything that wouldn't fit on the floor or on a shelf somewhere.

Rhodie was a special person in the Kid's life. She didn't walk so well. And when she did at all, she used a walking stick and did it very slowly. Coulda been arthritis. Coulda been she was too big to move much. She sat at the back of the store like a queen bee holding court. If you wanted a piece of baloney she'd slice it for you with that sharp butcher knife she kept near the box of crackers. And sometimes she'd slip you a piece of candy or a piece of cheese *for free!*

Dad used to call baloney "dog". For years he'd go into Rhodies and order "dog and crackers and a chunk of onion". In retrospect I guess Rhodie was like everybody's mom. Sitting back there. Not smiling. But still you knew she was your friend. The Kid knew instinctively that she was his buddy. Whenever he went into the store he made a beeline over to see Rhodie. Perhaps it was his Pavlovian conditioning to the treats he came to expect. He liked Rhodie. A lot.

There actually was only one downtown street in Puryear, but it was like a two-in-one. One strip was on the east side of the railroad tracks and the other was on the other side of the tracks. With a big dirt parking area on the Rhodies' side. Early strip mall.

Rhodies' front porch ran across four or five other stores all the way up to the cross street. The porch, or walkway, if you want to be sophisticated and call it that, was made out of rough unpainted wood. The stores, including Rhodies, had half-assed whitewash facades and, it seemed to the Kid, lots of metal signs advertising Coca Cola, Prince Albert Tobacco, Dr. Pepper, Hadacol and just about anything else there was in the world worth a damn. There was something special about those signs.

On a lucky Saturday night there'd be a tent pitched smack in the middle of Rhodies' dirt-paved parking lot with a picture show inside. They had electricity and everything in Puryear. It was the magic of electricity that changed life from humdrum happiness to pitch fever fun. Somebody would run a line from Rhodies to the other side of the parking lot under one of the big trees between her place and the railroad track. Then they'd put up this big army tent. The same kind of tent they used to put up for revival meetings which they also had a lot of in Rhodies' parking lot. Then they'd put wooden folding chairs inside in rows, facing the front. They'd set up a table in the middle of the center aisle. The projector went there. They'd put a couple of electric lights in there and send out the call.

For a nickel or a dime everybody in Puryear and environs was invited to see a moving picture show. Didn't matter what the subject was the crowd didn't vary according to matter. Whatever it was, was a hoot. For the adults this would be a welcome break from the backbreaking work of farming and homemaking. Everybody happily looked forward to it.

Until Sam Garrett made a sudden appearance in the rearview mirror.

Until drunken Sam Garrett came along.

A hidden time bomb whose cosmic purpose that night was to demonstrate how a single moment in time can reverberate, groping out in ever-widening ripples until every generation for the next hundred and fifty years has been poisoned by its acid-covered fingers.

Sam Garrett lived in Murray, Kentucky, which is located twenty-two miles north of Paris, Tennessee. "On the night in question" he had been pulled over by the Henry County Sheriff's Department for drunk driving. He was pulled over because he was having obvious problems keeping his car under control. But Sam Garrett was a good old boy and the sheriff said, "If you'll promise not to drink anymore tonight and that you'll drive yourself home directly from here I'll let you go. But you've got to go straight home."

Sam Garrett promised and was released, a catapult launching a jet plane from an aircraft carrier. He shot down U.S. 641 like a bullet. Sam Garrett was bent on keeping his word. Even through the alcoholic fog he could see how lucky he'd been.

Straight home. Nothing would keep him from his promise. Straight home. Arrow straight.

Straight through that pickup truck carrying those six Moody people on their way to a gala Saturday night in Puryear.

Straight through. Splattering their lives on the walls of eternity with blood that would never come off.

It took seconds.

To kill mom.

The impact popped the passenger door of the truck open. Mom's head was thrown to the side. The passenger slammed back and broke her neck. She was dead.

Suddenly the Kid was thrown into the middle of total confusion. The truck was on fire. Dad was somewhere yelling. He pulled the Kid out of the truck and Jacky and Peggy and Ronald and mom. They were all safe, he prayed. Safe.

"Let them all be safe, God."

"God. God. God."

"Let my family be all alright."

"Anything you want from me, God."

"Just let them be okay!"

The cries of that wounded man. A pitifully powerless howl of diminishing hope as he realized his family was no more.

God didn't listen that night. Or any of the other nights after that. God was too busy, I guess, to fuck with a poor dirt farmer's family who had nothing to offer the world except the skin off its back from the sun.

Yessir. God didn't give a good goddamn that night in nineteen-forty-seven. And if the Kid ever gets a chance he's gonna tell Him or Her or It — and he would so like there to be one — what he thinks of His eye being on the sparrow while the Kid's mom got crushed like a fucking bug by a drunk who kissed a sheriff's ass and got sent home with a friendly pat.

Ruby Gordon Sutton Moody died a totally unnecessary death that night. She never reached her twenty-seventh birthday. Hell, she never saw Ronald potty trained or the Kid and Jacky learn to read or Peggy grow into the beautiful woman who was, at a glance, her mother's daughter.

For years afterward the Kid had vengeance in his heart. When he grew up he was gonna hunt that Sam Garrett down and kill the son-of-a-bitch. Wherever he found him. Anyway he could. Outrage boiled up inside him whenever he heard that name mentioned. How dare they let him kill mom and not do anything about it! But he was cheated again. Sam Garrett died a natural death while the Kid was still in his teens.

Peggy was hurt. She had a broken arm. Ronald had a broken wrist. Dad had what looked, to the three year old Kid, like a hole in the right center of his forehead like somebody had shot him there with a Roy Rogers gun. The only scars Jacky and the Kid would have from that accident would be in their psyches which would guide their bodies slowly into self-destruction over the next few decades and deprive them for the rest of their lives of the sweet sense of home that they saw everywhere else.

Life got to be confusing after the accident. The next time he saw mom was at Aunt Louise's house. Lying in a casket. Quiet. Sleeping. She wouldn't wake up. She wouldn't look at him. She wouldn't talk to him. She just lay there in that casket like she was too tired to get up again. And all the flowers.

The Kid almost puked from the oppressive scent of the flowers around the room where mom was lying in the casket and later in the church where the funeral was held. For the rest of his life the smell of the blossoms of cut flowers would send him reeling to mom's casket. That odor that sucked the oxygen out of the air and transformed him into a three year old again. Confused and confounded by death. Again.

In later years the Kid would wonder which was worse: mom dying and taking off on him or the sympathetic clucking of all those relatives and friends and strangers while mom was laid out and being funeralized. Except for the fact that mom refused to talk to him or yell at him anymore, that strange behavior by adults toward him told him more than words could have that there was something bad happening in his life.

Where Kiddies Fly

Grandmother Sutton had, ostensibly, shooed the Kid and Jacky out back to fetch kindling wood for the cookstove. What she really wanted was a couple of minutes away from those two poor little orphans whose next of kin were banshees.

They raced each other to the woodpile on the far side of the lot where junk wood was piled higher than either one of them. Jacky bent over and started picking up small pieces of wood that would help grandmother. The Kid grabbed a foot-long piece of wood and whacked Jacky on the head with it. "That's my job," he yelled.

Jacky grabbed his head and started screaming. The offending piece of wood had a bent rusty nail sticking out the end. The bent rusty nail had left a trail of blood flowing down from the center of Jacky's head to his face.

Never mind that the Kid was two years younger than Jacky; he was ancient by comparison in temperament. The Kid had learned to throw tantrums like an adult when he was very young. Jacky was basically a nice guy. He'd grow up to get along except when it came to affairs of the heart and of cash. The Kid would spend his whole life feeling pissed off about one thing or the other.

When he was four years old, which was his age at the woodpile, he was pissed off primarily for one of two reasons: when someone told him "no", and when he wasn't in charge. The bang on Jacky's head arose from the "not in charge" mode. Jacky ran back to the house to tell grandmother. The Kid ran back to soften the damage as much as he could, and, if he was really lucky, to avoid a switching from a peach tree branch.

By the time grandmother had examined the wound, stanched the bleeding, and calmed Jacky, she was not up to forgiving the Kid for his reasoning, no matter how painfully honest it was. "He made me mad and I hit him. He made me mad and I hit him. And I'm proud of it." The peach tree branch that afternoon was strong and left a lingering sting.

The Moodys lived on the Hervie Hancock place. There was a big dairy barn and feedlot for the cows dad milked for Hervie. And the fields: watermelons, sweet potatoes, tobacco and tomatoes. As young as they were the Kid and Jacky would help set out sweet potato and tobacco slips in the spring; bending over to place the slips just so far apart until their backs felt like a hayloft dance floor after a Hank Williams concert. They helped, whenever dad called on them, in the fields and the barn and the lot.

The fact that their job was mostly twice done — once by them and once again by dad — was a credit to the fact that dad didn't give up on their willingness to contribute to the common good.

Ruby Gordon Moody had been killed in an auto accident less than a year ago. That was a still an unresolved family problem. The Moody family that summer consisted of Connie Taylor Moody, thirty-one, the father; Peggy Joyce Moody, nine, probably the most sensible of the clan, who had her hands full helping to take care of young Ronald Henry Moody, one; Jacky Royce Moody, six, mostly affable but subject to seizures of extreme stubbornness, as were most members of the family, and petulance; and the Kid, four, who was a born again brat.

22

Oh, yes, then there was Henry Elmore Sutton, the granddaddy who didn't get to say very much because he was there with Nell Sutton, the grandmother who did all the family thinking and talking and decision making, thank you very much. At least on the surface anyhow.

The two of them had gone up to Detroit several years earlier to make their retirement money and come home to Henry County, Tennessee on a featherbed of comfort for the rest of their lives. Mom's death blasted that dream all to hell. They came back to Tennessee for the funeral and stayed on to take care of us kids and otherwise help dad return to some semblance of normalcy as head of household and breadwinner.

He never did and they left, mostly because dad and grandmother couldn't get along, but in the summer of nineteen-forty-seven they were there.

The Kid didn't remember much about what granddaddy did around the house. He supposed he helped out in the fields, for he'd been a farmer most of his life, having raised six kids on a farm before he'd turned to carpentry. And he probably helped with the milking. And the gardening. And whatever chores grandmother had for him.

That was the "we" that summer. Grandmother giving the kids doses of castor oil at the first hint of a headache or tummy ache. We didn't get sick very often and if you've ever been dosed with castor oil you'd understand perfectly why any sane human being, regardless of age, would strive for perfection of health symptoms. "No, Grandmother, I don't have a headache. I've been too close to the stove and got too hot. No, I don't need any medicine 'cause I'm not sick. I feel good. Did I say I was going to lie down? No. No. I'm on my way out

23

to play with Jacky. I feel good, Grandmother. I feel so good."

The castor oil wasn't a lot of help the time the cow stomped on the Kid's right foot. Right on top of the instep. In the dairy barn on the concrete floor. Jesus did that hurt. The foot was flatter 'n a fritter for days, not to mention the fact that it carried a very clear imprint of a cow's hoof. And she looked so loving, staring at him with those big mooney eyes as she twitched a couple of flies off her back with her tail and looked to get rid of a pest of a different kind with a well-placed step.

The dairy barn was interesting. It had concrete floors for ease of cleaning. It had running water to facilitate cleaning all the stuff that's gotta be cleaned and kept clean when you sell milk on a medium-to-large scale like dad and Hervie Hancock were doing. I suspect the difference in the care taken with cleanliness is that it's easier to eat one five gallon can of bad milk than ten cans. One you can feed to the hogs. Ten cans is too expensive to let happen.

Dad and granddaddy and neighbors helped put in the crops. Hervie Hancock came around pretty often, to keep an eye on dad methinks. Hervie owned a lot of land in Henry County. He was a true white massuh who treated his sharecroppers kindly, if not generously, much like on the old Deep South plantations owned by kindly whites. Young as the Kid was he remembered Hervie pressing a quarter into his little hand every time he came by to survey his fiefdom.

Jacky was a glutton for most of his life. Grandmother always fixed a big farm breakfast of gravy and eggs and bacon and biscuits and molasses and butter. Jacky was the first one to sit down and start piling food on his plate. If, while he was eating, he saw someone else start to take something he thought he might want more of when he'd finished what he had, he'd call them down on it. "Don't eat that, I might want some more when I'm done with this."

Whether from the trauma of mom's murder or what, Jacky, for months after her death, would stuff himself until he had to puke. Then he'd run outside, puke, come back inside and start all over again. God, we were a sad lot that summer.

And that was the best summer we had after she left us.

Mom's death didn't even slow the Kid down. He drove grandmother to distraction. One day she walked into the kitchen to find sugar poured over everything. Five pounds of sugar dumped over the table, the stove, the floor, the cabinets. Everything!

Where it had gotten wet it had turned to syrup, sticking everything to everything else. The Kid didn't have any ulterior motive, though. He'd run into the kitchen to get a drink of water from the water bucket. As he raised the dipper to his lips, a brand new unopened bag of sugar sitting on the cabinet caught his eye. He found a knife.

Jacky would turn out to be the most stubborn. Some say in the summer of nineteen-forty-seven that he perfected it. Grandmother would tell Jacky to do something. Anything. "No. I'm mad and I ain't gonna do it." And he wouldn't. She or dad or God hisself coulda beat that boy til his eyes bugged out and he wouldn't have done it. Had to let him cool off first. Then he might.

The Kid and Jacky were both stubborn as mules. But that was one contest the Kid lost out big time. Jacky Royce would die at age fifty-five in aching isolation because he was too stubborn to make the trek back to people who loved him.

The one thing about the Kid that wasn't mean that summer was the dream that wouldn't go away. Every single night for more than a year he dreamt he was in an open field, like a wheat field, running, running when suddenly something ominously fearful began to chase him. He ran faster and faster, so fast that he was breathing his own saliva causing his nose to sting like he'd been pushed underwater for too long. And faster and faster. And every time he'd glance over his shoulder the fearful thing was gaining. Until suddenly it leaped. And he'd wake up.

After Jacky had died he wondered if he had had dreams, too, after mom got killed.

The crops came in. A field full of tomatoes for the market and also perfect hand grenades for war with Jacky as the two stood in the middle of the patch taking a bite out of one before blasting the brother with it.

Ripe watermelons laying all around begging for two little kids to run down the road, pick one up, smash it on the ground and reach in with eager fists to grab the sweet "heart" of its meat.

And the sweet potatoes which were as hard to harvest as they were to set out. Filling those tall round crates. Day after day after day. Was no fun. Did not make wonderful memories. Did make pain and agony, even though the kids didn't put out half the work they thought they did. They spent as much time playing around the

26

edges of the fields as they did digging in the fields, maybe more. Probably more.

Rena Mae used to visit us at the Hancock place. The Kid walked with her a hundred times on those afternoon sojourns from the time he was four. Up the road past the house where the boy who'd been in Boliver [West Tennessee State (mental) Hospital] lived. Which was kinda scary, 'cause everybody said the boy was crazy and they wouldn't be surprised at anything he might do to somebody if his parents ever let him slip through their hands and escape into the neighborhood.

All the Kid knew was that something so fearsome would happen to him if that boy ever caught him that it would be too horrible a tale to tell. *Is he looking at me? He IS looking at me! He's walking over this way. He's going to get me. He's going to get me. He's going to get me!* His soul screamed for him to get out of there and Rena Mae acted as if nothing was happening. She never once picked up her pace. She never once bent over and picked up a big rock to defend them with. Just kept on going like nothing was wrong while the Kid was quaking with dread.

Grownups talked about him a lot whenever they got together of a night on somebody's front porch and passed the time with conversation. "I hear tell that boy's bad crazy. 'Course you can't tell by lookin'. He seems like he's alright when somethin' sets 'im off.

Real crazy. Like he ain't got a brain in his head. Jumping up and down. Froth out his mouth. Don't know where he is or what he's doing. And he'd been that way since he was knee-high. Just went crazy one day. Why, he'll wake up, they say, and act like nothin' has happened. When he's not crazy he's just as likeable as you'd ever want to meet."

There were a lot of good times that summer. Like the Sunday mom's siblings came for the day: Aunt Margaret and Uncle Telous, Uncle Pete and Aunt Betty, Aunt Maxine and Uncle Ambry, Uncle J and Aunt Lillian. And then there was Uncle Sam and Aunt Naomi. Grandmother cooked dinner. Then they gathered in the front yard to let the food settle. Talking. About family and hopes and mom's death. And how was Connie getting along. And the kids. And grandmother and granddaddy.

Grandmother later said Jacky and the Kid were so rough with the adult men that they hurt their backs by jumping all over them. A four year old and a six year old to blame for injuries to adult males in their twenties. Apparently because they were the devil's seed or something equally sinister. Peggy was never included, I suppose, because she was a girl and seen by grandmother through different eyes. And Ronald? I don't know why he never got shot down for hitting someone or wiggling too much or biting or crying, but he didn't. He turned out to be grandmother's favorite perhaps because he didn't hurt her grownup children, therefore he wasn't all bad.

There were several Sundays like that over the summer of forty-seven. Treasures.

But those good times were coming to an end, to be replaced by other, much different, times. Grandmother and dad got into it once too often. They had never liked each other. Grandmother thought mom way too good to be married to trash like Connie Moody. Dad thought grandmother was a nosey old bitch trying to run his life. They finally called it quits. Grandmother would say "without as much as a thank you after all we'd done for him and you kids."

Grandmother and granddaddy moved to Paris where granddaddy would spend several years buying rundown houses, living in them while he fixed them up, then selling them and moving on to another. Dad would replace grandmother with a parade of babysitter types none of whom had her disciplinarian resolve.

And Home Fires Burn Low

Confusion mutated into chaos after grandmother and grandfather left. Actually I should say since grandmother left because granddaddy never caused any trouble for anybody anyhow so he can't be counted in the fun-meter measurement of good ole but doddering times.

The Kid and Jacky were happy. With no one to yell at them and whale on their butts and maintain some sense of discipline, they were off on the ride of their lives. The Kid would think up the mischief and Jacky would tag along. They could now add the house proper to their playground, starting with peeing contests in the early morning. Jacky would jump out of bed and run slamming through the screen door to the porch where another day promised more great adventures. The Kid peed at him through the screen, mostly stinking up the screen. Not to be outdone Jacky would pull out his little pecker and pee an arch back into the house.

The slamming doors and the giggling boys attracted some attention. Sometimes dad would whomp up on one or both their butts, but usually it was just the babysitter who didn't warrant even a one on a scale of ten. These guys were pros. A slap or two on the cheek of rump or face was nothing compared to what grandmother had dished out. Or before her, mom. Besides, who cared as long as they were having fun! What it *was* was Disneyland. Lordy! Lordy! What fun those boys had.

Anarchy grew.

Grandmother said one of the reasons granddaddy and she left was because dad went back to drinking and carousing, stepping out with women, going to beer gardens and paying less and less attention to the farm and the family. "Me and Elmore wasn't about to do his work for him. I don't care if he was Ruby's husband. The only reason we stayed as long as we did was for the kids. But finally we just couldn't take it any longer so we moved out and still kept hoping he'd shape up and get his life back in order for the sake of you kids, if not for hisself."

The fact was dad was fucking up royally. Hervie Hancock visited ever more often to try to keep a rein on him. Of course, Peggy, Jacky, and the Kid loved that, for every visit meant another quarter. Alms for the poor orphaned Moody kids who didn't give a shit about his motivation as long as it meant some money in their palms.

The whole bunch was not so quietly coming apart at the seams. One night a rat ran up onto the bed where Peggy was sleeping and bit her on the nose. A goddamn rat bit her on the face! On the same bed where mom had stood the Kid the night she dressed him for her death dance.

That poor girl was scared out of her mind. Inconsolable. She screamed for hours, seemed like. She'd open her mouth to say something and the only thing that would come out was more scream or a hard-packed pocket of air which had outrun its scream somewhere between the pit of her soul and her voice box.

She was a mess for weeks afterward. Afraid to go to sleep. And when she finally got too tired to stay awake and search for rats, she'd put her head under a pillow and cry herself to sleep. Dad put out rat traps and poison, but she wouldn't be comforted. Goddamn rats. Goddamn vermin of all kinds. Goddamn.

Jacky was in first grade in nineteen-forty-eight. Peggy was in third. They rode the bus to Puryear School, a long red-brick building with a million windows where all the kids in the whole county around there went. First grade to twelve. Never mind kindergarten; there wudn't any.

Jacky's teacher was Miss Pillow, the same first grade teacher Peggy had and the same first grade teacher the Kid would have two years from now. I think Peggy's teacher was Miz Gallimore but I'm not for sure. I do remember she had a face like a hawk. That woman looked like she'd swoop down on you and take you to her nest for lunch if you didn't watch yourself. Her looks belied her good disposition as the Kid discovered when Peggy used to take him to class with her once in awhile.

The teacher and other students would pet him all day and he luxuriated in that even if he was like a nice kitty-cat or teddy-bear. The girls gave him lots and lots of attention. Even one or two of the boys would come up during the day and chuck him on the shoulder, although they weren't nearly as sincere as the wannabe mommas. Miz Gallimore sat him on an upended sweet potato hamper over near a window by Peggy's desk where she was handy in case he needed her or got too loud, as he was wont to do. Peggy gave him pencil and paper to keep him quiet and out of trouble.

The best of all things that happened to the Kid was he fell in love with Linda Lou Hart, one of Peggy's friends. The kid would fall in love a lot during the next half century, but never harder or more profoundly than with Linda Lou. She was beautiful, the most beautiful third-grader there ever had been. She was friendly. She'd walk over and talk to him several times during the day with that sunshiny smile.

32

The Kid would remain smitten by her until he died. Every time he'd think about her his heart would warm up and his soul would smile. If he'd had any sense back then when he was four and if he'd been Chinese he'd gotten engaged to her right then so she wouldn't have run off with some other guy and got married and had kids. He would have made her happier than she could have ever dreamed happy was. He was her guy.

Peggy had a blue and white girls bicycle she used to ride up and down the hill. All the roads off U.S. 641 were gravel roads which was good because when it rained cars and trucks wouldn't get stuck in a foot-and-a-half deep sinkhole. One day Peggy Joyce was riding lickety-split down the hill as fast as her legs would propel her. Peggy's bicycle hit some loose gravel causing her to lose her balance. Bike and girl skidded forever, it seemed, on that gravel before they stopped.

Peggy's legs and arms were torn up. They looked like raw hamburger meat. We could hear Peggy screaming down there where she was sitting on the side of the road bleeding and hurting. Dad came running from the barn. The Kid would never forget the abject pain on Peggy's face as she silently pleaded for help to end her nightmare. Nobody went to the doctor those days unless they were dying. Salves were applied and bandages torn from old sheets put to use.

Life sometimes looks upside down and inside out when you're four years old and trying to make sense of a world that is nothing like it was when you were three. I suspect one of the other reasons dad's in-laws took a hike from the Hancock place was because of dad's romancing Annie Catherine Bray.

Annie Catherine was a divorcee who lived on the other side of Puryear with her mom and dad and daughter Zora Ann. Zora Ann was a year older than the Kid. I don't know how they met or where or when except that it wasn't long enough in grandmother's lexicon to be considered a decent interval after mom's murder.

Dad started going out at night once in awhile. Then more frequently until he was gone just about every night of the week, it seemed. And that's about when the farm and the kids started playing second fiddle to his obsessive escapes from a world that had killed him already, except for stopping his damn heart.

Housekeeping at the Hancock place was a day job. Somebody to cook and clean and half-ass watch after the kids until dad got home from the fields. Then it was scrambling to find someplace for the kids to go after dark. I don't remember where Peggy and Ronald would go; I suspect they'd visit Betty Jo Valentine, Peggy's friend, and her family. Bernice, Betty Jo's mom, loved Peggy and the whole family was great, except for the Pete Valentine bogeyman.

Dad and Annie Catherine would drop off Jacky and the Kid at the house of those colored people who lived at the corner of Pete Valentine Road and U.S. 641. Dad was always solicitous as he prepared his getaway. "Now you kids sure you'll be alright? I won't leave you unless it's okay with you."

Being without their father at night tacked onto being without their mom day and night was unsettling for awhile. Oh, they loved their sitters, but every time that old car backed out of that dirt yard Jacky and the Kid knew full well they were being abandoned, even if they did recover quickly.

34

Annie Catherine's fare-thee-well was a promise. "If y'all be good and nice for these folks I'll get your daddy to bring you back something special." Then she'd hug us and kiss us and walk over to the car that dad had somehow come up with since mom's murder. They'd turn from the kids, each would open his/her car door and kind of spring in with a flourish, slam the door and be off to the races. To get drunk and laid.

At the colored family's house Jacky and the Kid always had a wonderful time, although the mom killed some of the fun when she made her three year old daughter stop taking off her panties so the Kid could satisfy his curiosity and see how she was made different from Jacky and him. A four year old lothario.

Needless to say, metamorphosis was ever present at the Moody house. The family structure was not very slowly being smashed to smithereens. Family activities became a thing of the past. Meals were increasingly for kids and housekeepers only. Farm work became a concept used ever more infrequently in dad's life. Questions of who we were became what will happen to us. Even in four and six and nine year old minds.

The kids kept him bothered about how he was screwing up everybody's life when all he meant to screw up was his own which he proclaimed loudly and at length every time he came home drunk. "I don't even want to go on," he'd moan as tears tumbled from his drunken eyes and he'd grab us kids in a bear hug and fumigate us. "What's the use?"

Some of our aunts and uncles were concerned about what was happening to the kids while dad was gallivanting around the country. On at least two different occasions Uncle Pete drove out when dad was home to try to convince him to straighten up, or, if he was bound to kill himself, to give the kids up and give them a chance which they sure as hell weren't getting with him acting like he was. Dad would agree if he was sober and would try to start a fight if he wasn't.

"Ain't nobody gonna talk to Connie Moody like that," he'd say. "Connie Moody will by god take care of Connie Moody's kids. And I'll kill the first sumbitch that tries to take my kids away from me. My kids is all in the world I've got left, Pete. I ain't givin' 'em up." Uncle Pete would drive away.

Pete Valentine's dad and mom lived within spitting distance across the road from us. In the interest of togetherness, Pete sent a big crew up to his parents' house one day and had them roll the house down the hill next to Pete's house. On logs! The Kid watched 'em.

It was a crackerbox house. Four rooms with a tin roof. Clapboard siding painted white. A porch ran all the way across the front, its roof supported by wooden posts. Still, it was bigger than your average school lunch bucket. All it took was one day. They rolled it across the road through our pasture and feedlot and down the hill. They just kept putting big-ass logs in front of it and pulling it with a couple teams of mules and "voila"!

Sometimes Rena Mae would come over and take the kids visiting. Peggy and Ronald seemed like creatures from another planet to Jacky and the Kid. They were quiet and well-behaved if you didn't count Ronald's crying jags. You hardly even knew they were around when grownups were sitting on the porch or in the shaded living room of a summer afternoon.

The Kid could feel the red clay gravel crunching under his bare feet as he bounced along, consciously oblivious to the oppression of his own world which was slowly but inexorably collapsing about him.

One day dad had the housekeeper watch the kids for several days. They stayed home. At the Hancock place. Three or four days later he brought hisself home a bride. "Annie Catherine is going to be living with us from now on kids. She already loves you and I know you'll love her too. She won't ever replace your mom, but she'll be here to help take care of you."

And Zora Ann.

And Zora Ann.

Jacky and the Kid had thought they were going to love having Zora Ann in the family. She was sandwiched between them age wise and seemed like a playful enough person. It'd be like a playground.

What they hadn't counted on was that Zora Ann was a crybaby and went bawling to her mother every time she wanted to get even with the Kid or Jacky. Every single time Zora Ann ran to her mom and told on them they'd get punished. Every goddamn thing Zora Ann told Annie Catherine Annie Catherine believed and acted accordingly with birch and peach and much yelling and screeching.

Zora Ann was not any fun. They didn't like her. They didn't want her around them getting them into trouble a dozen times a day. And they didn't want her around vacuuming all the love and favors Annie Catherine had to give.

Dad continued to lose his taste for hard work. And then we got kicked off Mr. Hancock's farm because he didn't run a charity ward.

Bulls and Butcher Knives

The Kid raced into the house on the heels of his brother Jacky and slammed the front door behind him. He ran to the window and sagged against the sill panting, looking for signs that they'd followed them to the house. The neighbor kids with the butcher knives. Both slumped in relief when they realized they had survived one more assault.

They were crazy. Flat out fucking crazy. Why else would they come running maniacally from all directions whenever little kids walked by. Waving big-ass butcher knives way above their heads, trying to slash anybody who was smaller than they were? Why else? They had to be crazy.

All the Kid knew was that Jacky and he ran faster than they'd ever run before every time they were pursued by them. One of the attackers was a giant. He must have been ten or twelve years old. Surely only a miracle kept him from overtaking one of the two. After all the Kid was only five and Jacky seven. And they both thought they were pretty tough hombres until they ran into the kids from the corner. Now they were afraid to go out of their front yard. Which was a shame because there was a whole new world to explore, if they could only get to it.

The Moody's had gone to the city. Paris, Tennessee. Population eight thousand and change.

Dad's ambition to work had steadily deteriorated since mom got killed in that car wreck two years ago, so he'd lost his share of the Hancock farm off U.S. 641. Part of that share was a place to live for himself and his new wife Annie Catherine Bray Moody and his kids Peggy Joyce, Jacky Royce, the Kid, Ronald Henry and her kid

Zora Ann Bray. And the other thing, Annie Catherine wasn't about to be a slave to no damned farm, especially one where dad had lived in bliss with mom until the drunk man did her in.

The house in Paris was actually half a house. The owner, a bachelor in his sixties, lived in the smaller upstairs while the Moody clan moved into the bigger downstairs. This was modern living. Running water in the house! A kerosene stove! With one of those big glass bottles of coal oil, about the size of a drinking fountain water bottle, upended on the right side of the porcelain covered stove. No more cutting wood or, for the kids relaxing pleasure, totin' wood for the cookstove. And an electric refrigerator! Electric anything! Electric everything! Electric lights! Flick a switch and the whole world blossomed into some kind of yellowish orange phantasm.

It was in the Paris house the Kid saw his first stick of margarine. Real butter was all he'd ever eaten on the farm and the farm was all he'd ever known until he moved into the town house. The first time was the best. Annie Catherine took a package of white gunk out of the refrigerator and slapped it into a bowl; dumped some yellow stuff from a little package on top of it and then mixed it all up so it was kinda yellow and not quite so pale. She then smoothed it all over in a rounded mound just like butter, except butter that had stayed in the sunshine too long. It tasted like butter-flavored lard that didn't have a lot of flavor to it.

It was also where he first saw dad and Annie Catherine nekkid in bed together. Even though he couldn't see everything he knew they were nekkid 'cause they didn't have anything on the arms or shoulders. Wudn't that hard to figure out. But it did look like it was

39

kinda silly to sleep without any clothes on when it got so chilly at night.

It was a big two-storied house that sat on top of a hill just west of the railroad tracks in northwest Paris. On a gravel road. There was a big tree in the front yard down by the pasture. This was a pasture which was the second scariest thing about that neighborhood where the Kid was concerned. A white-faced bull. The pasture ran next to the yard of the house. It was also across the road from the crazy kids' house.

The first time the Kid and Jacky met the bull they were running away from the knife-wielding crazy kids. It was a shortcut to their house so they jumped over the fence and started running through the field to their front yard. About halfway over the shouts of their pursuers they heard something that sounded like a snort. You know, like a bull snorting.

One glance and they just about shit their britches. It wasn't bad enough that a bunch of crazy kids intent on slitting their throats were chasing them from behind. No. Now out of left field comes the thundering hoofbeats of a damn bull that's as big as a house with guest rooms.

Oh, shit! Lungs that couldn't breathe anymore managed. Legs that had dropped off halfway back kept moving. Somehow. Somehow. They made it to the fence. Pulled themselves to the top strand, mindless of the fact that it was barbed wire, and tumbled over into their yard and stumbled onto their feet and ran, as fast as they could, to their front door.

Only after they were safely inside did they look back and laugh. "Hey Jacky look. Look out there in the pasture at them boys now. Look at 'em. They're scared of that bull, Jack." Having lost his first prey, the bull saw other young meat coming up the hill toward the yard. He never missed a beat as he swerved and thundered after the crazy kids who now were yelling a different tune. "The goddamn bull is coming this way! Get out of here! Get out of here! Run, goddammit! Get out of here!" They obviously were every bit as spooked by that white-faced bull as Jacky and the Kid had been.

From then on the recurring dilemma the Moody kids had to face every time they went past the crazy kids' house was whether to chance the butcher knives and run the long way home down the road and up the hill to the front porch or chance the horns and run through the pasture to the side yard which was almost at their doorway.

The miracle was that neither the boys nor the bull ever caught up with them. Years later Jacky said he met up with the big kid and cussed him out for scaring his brother and him so badly. Since the big bully didn't have his butcher knife with him, Jacky said he just stood there and took it until he was finished then turned around and walked away.

The Kid didn't know what dad was doing for a living while they lived in Paris. He'd only ever known him as a farmer and thought he was probably going off every day to work on a farm somewhere. Later, he figured he was probably working any kind of job he could get. Anything to make enough money to buy food and beer and pay the rent, if there was enough left over.

The Kid had no memory of Peggy and Ronald being in the house on the hill. He figured they probably visited grandmother and granddaddy a couple of miles on the other side of town.

A lot.

41

For very long periods of time. Otherwise, he should remember something. He remembered Zora Ann, for god's sake.

Still, there was fun to be had on the hill. In addition to running in terror from bulls and boys. One of the favorite things for the Kid and Jacky to do was see who could jump from the higher limb on the big tree in the front yard by the pasture. They'd start out on the bottom limbs which they had to shinny up four or five feet to, then get daring. The Kid won most of the time. Because the Kid didn't give a shit whether he broke his neck as long as he won. He can remember several times when his head rang like a bell when he hit the ground from an upper branch. Just like a bell, except that a bell probably didn't have that kind of headache. Day after day after day.

Dad loved his beer-drinking country music and his beer drinking. One morning the cops came to the house and said something to Annie Catherine. She started crying, shoved us kids aside — Zora Ann, Jacky and the Kid — and started rummaging through a cedar chest.

"Whatchoo lookin' for, Catherine?"

"I'm looking for Zora Ann's savings bonds, Kid. They took your daddy to jail last night and I gotta bail him out. And I ain't got no money except them savings bonds. I don't know what I'm gonna do with Connie Moody, Kid. I know he's your daddy and I love him, but I swear I can't do anything with him. What am I gonna do with him?" She grabbed the Kid as tears ran down her face into his hair.

She found the bonds and dad. Annie Catherine wasn't ready for a quiet reunion and dad wasn't ready to take any guff off anybody, so the trip home was a cacophony for two lovers in the front seat of a car winding its way through the streets of Paris.

"Goddamn it, Connie! I can't live like this! I swear if you don't stop this I'm gonna pack up and leave you. I can't stand it anymore." Her voice found new energy and volume with each word until it reached a crescendo that would have brought the courthouse down if the courthouse coulda been brought down by a shrill scream emptying itself pitifully in the sunlit morning air.

"If you don't like it, you can leave any goddamn time you want to. I ain't got no chains on you. And I ain't asking you to stay. If you don't like it go! Get outta here. I don't need you. And I definitely ain't gonna stand for your sass. So, if you wanna go, get your stuff and get out. Don't let the door hit you in the ass, Catherine. Me and the kids got along before you came and we'll be just fine after you leave. Connie Moody don't need you or any other whore. If you want to stay, then shut up!"

Dad and Annie Catherine fought a lot for all the years they were together. Later the Kid would hear that dad was pimping for her. Whether it was true or not, the Kid knew it could have been true. He mostly felt sad. It wasn't like his moral sensibilities had been offended. They hadn't been. It was sad because he knew if it was true it was almost certainly what had driven dad and her apart for the last and final time.

Back home from jail, at the homestead on the hillside, dad and Annie Catherine got out of the car, walked into the house, looked at each other for a minute, and broke into a hug which transmogrified into a grope which translated itself into orders, "All kids outside. Right now! We've got stuff to talk about. Don't nobody even try to get in until we have time to straighten this out. You hear?!"

The Kid didn't have a watch on him, but his belly told him it was way after dinner by the time they'd worked things out. Which must have been hard work, he figured, from the shape they were in by the time they unlocked the door.

One afternoon dad pulled into a little grocery store for cigarettes. Everybody piled out and went inside. The Kid made his usual rounds looking for the best of the goodies and lusting for a dozen of the crème de la crème. But nooooo, nobody offered to buy him any of that wonderful flat coconut candy, the stuff that came in multicolored layers. Nobody offered to buy him jackshit. There obviously was only one thing left for him to do if he were to survive the day.

The Kid grabbed the bag of candy and went out to the car where he promptly tore it open and started eating before anybody could take it away from him. And ate. Until a policeman came over and opened the passenger side of the car, looked at the Kid, and asked, "Did you steal this candy, kid?"

The Kid just looked at that huge man whom he was sure would pinch his head off without even trying hard if he had a mind to. Just looked. With his mouth hanging open. The cop pulled the Kid out of the car. "Okay, kid, I guess I'll just have to take you to jail." And dragged him over to his police car and onto the back seat. The Kid was so scared his knees were knocking together. He knew his life was over at the age of five.

Just as the cop was going around to get in behind the steering wheel, dad came out. "What's going on, officer?" he asked, his face as innocent as a baby's behind.

"Caught this boy stealing candy from the store in there. You know him?"

"Don't think so. Let me have a closer look at 'im. Well, now he does look a little like the Kid. Could be. Except the Kid wouldn't go around stealing candy off store shelves. Are you the Kid?" The Kid nodded desperately. He was too frightened to speak.

"Tell you what, officer. Let him go with me this once and I'll make sure he never does anything like that again."

"Okay, but you better make sure he understands stealing is serious business. Do you understand that, son?" The Kid nodded desperately. "Okay, you can get out then and go with your dad." Sweeter words were never spoken.

Only one other time did dad threaten the Kid with a cop. And that wasn't too long afterwards. Dad had taken the Kid with him in the car up to the poolroom where dad liked to go drink beer sometimes. After an hour or two the Kid got tired and went back to the car. The cars were parked diagonally with their right front tire against the curb. After the Kid opened the passenger side door, but before he climbed in for his short summer's nap, he was struck by the urgent call of nature. *Kid, you gotta pee! Kid, you better pee before you pee your pants! Right now!*

Not being one to ignore the call of nature, the Kid grabbed his pecker and pointed it toward the juncture of the sidewalk and street just before it loosed its load of whatever was loosed whenever he had to go pee. In mid-pee, dad walked out of the poolroom, took one look and raised his hand toward somebody behind the Kid's back.

45

"Officer, there's somebody peeing on the street over here. Officer!" The Kid's head jerked back. Sure enough, there was a cop in a cruiser on the other side of the street. He pissed all over himself stuffing his urinary escape valve back into its closet of cloth. Dad looked again. "Guess I was mistaken officer. Nothing wrong as far as I can see." The Kid figured his unreasonable fear of cops arose from those two incidents that stuck with him his whole life long.

The kid felt cheated. It seemed like lots of things were not going his way. Mom had been killed in a car wreck in nineteen-forty-seven. The family had gotten kicked off the Hancock farm where dad had share-cropped because dad spent more time drinking corn than raising it. Home had deteriorated from a big comfortable farmhouse to a house they shared with the old man in Paris. From there to a claptrap house, with no electricity, over on Whitlock Road.

The house was actually made of unchinked logs. Weathered. Unpainted. Filled with cracks to let the wind freeze your butt off in the wintertime, but a great air conditioner in the summertime.

It had a roof of wooden shingles which did not cover all the holes. The front porch was small and collapsing in on itself. The back porch was huge and ran the entire backside of the house with a lot of dips and curves and places where you'd fall through the rotting wood if you weren't careful. The water well was in the middle of the back porch, surrounded by walls of wood which were in the process of returning to that from whence they came, that is, the earth. The back porch playground was a marvelous obstacle course. It was great fun if you didn't fall in. The miracle is that no kid's body was seriously broken during their tenure there.

The Kid's strongest memory of that old back porch would be of the screaming arguments between dad and Annie Catherine over the dispute of the day. The Kid and Jacky, playing on the back porch or in the backyard, agreed that those two were going to break up. It was clearly a matter of time. "What you gonna do, Jacky, when Catherine leaves? You gonna go with her or stay with dad?" "I'm gonna stay with dad." "Well, I'm not; I'm gonna go with Annie Catherine." "I like dad the best." "Nah, I like Catherine the best." They did split but not until half a dozen years later after Jacky and the Kid were long gone.

Peggy and Ronald had moved with the rest of the family there, except for Zora Ann, Annie Catherine's daughter from a previous marriage or a previous liaison or a previous immaculate conception.

Life had changed a lot for the Moody family by then. Dad was working over at the Whitlock sawmill when he felt like it which became less and less frequently.

There often wasn't enough food to feed the family. Dad had a twenty-two caliber rifle he took to the woods out back and shot rabbits and squirrels and birds and possums and anything else that moved. That was the meat they had most of the time. There was a big open fireplace in the combination living room and master bedroom where dad and Annie Catherine slept.

It had an iron hook from which was suspended a small kettle which was filled with beans, potatoes and onions and whatever food could be bought or found or stolen when there was some food to be bought or found or stolen. Dad called it slumgullion. The Kid remembered the white soup beans and potatoes flavored with onions and pepper. Forty-five years later the Kid and Jacky would reminisce fondly about the wonderful food dad cooked up in the kettle in the fireplace.

Annie Catherine fried dad's daily bag on the small kerosene stove in the tiny step-down kitchen which looked and felt like it would fall off into the gully behind the house if someone jumped up and down a little too hard. The Kid remembered standing by her side watching her fry possum one evening and seeing her cry as she watched it like a hawk because if it was burnt there was no second line of supper. The Kid adored Annie Catherine and she responded by often talking to him like he was a real person. "I don't know how long I can take this, Kid. I know Connie tries his best. But you know he's not over your momma and he won't ever get over her and as long as he's not over her he's going to keep on drinking and gettin' worse and one of these days there ain't gonna be nothin' in this house for any of us to eat. What we gonna do then, Kid?"

She shuddered with sobs as she stood there with those protruding eyes clouded by the disappointment that she'd married another no-good just like the first no-good, wearily waving the fork she held above the splattering possum's deep-fried remains.

When there was no money and no squirrels and rabbits or anything else to keep the wolf even kinda at bay, dad would pile the family into the car, cruise around back country and steal a meal. Lots of folk over by Whitlock woke up mornings missing a chicken or a sackful of corn or tomatoes or watermelons. If it was edible and it wasn't tied down and his family was hungry and he thought he could get away with it, dad would steal anything. But almost exclusively from colored folks because "who'd believe a nigger that white folks wuz stealin' from em? Ain't no goddamn way."

Even with the thievery, Annie Catherine's prediction of even harder food times came to pass. There came a time when there was no food at all in the log house. A time when there was no money for gas for the DeSoto. A time when the only recourse dad had to keep the Kid and

Jacky from starving was to take them for "visits" to family and friends.

Aunt Louise, his sister, would feed them and love them for a week or two at a time even though at the time she had three of her own.

The Watsons, friends who lived on the farm near the Hancock place, would feed them and love them for a week or two at a time. The Watson's kids were grown up and in their thirties by then, but they embraced the Moody boys with every bit of love they gave to each other.

On at least one of those occasions when the log house was foodless dad walked Jacky and the Kid several miles—the Kid thought they'd never get there—to the Watsons. "I've brought the boys here so they can at least eat. I know I've done wrong but I can't let 'em starve, so I'm asking you to let them stay here until I can get on my feet. I'm asking you. And I'm telling you I don't know if I'll be able to pay you, or, if I can, when."

"Connie, you know these boys are always welcome over here." Mr. Watson was the speaker. "And you're welcome here, too, anytime you're not drinking. You're welcome to eat supper and spend the night if you want to. You don't ever have to ask for these children."

"I'll be back for them soon as I can." Dad walked down the hill away from the house and up the road north toward Puryear. On his way he would walk over the spot in the pavement where his wife was killed by a drunk driver less than two years before. Where that drunk driver smashed all of Connie Moody's dreams to smithereens. The Kid and Jacky and the Watsons watched quietly as dad walked away. As he disappeared around the curve.

The Kid would remember baby Ronald—he couldn't have been even two years old—playing with Jacky and the Kid, and perhaps Peggy, with Peggy's bicycle out in the front yard of the log house. They turned the bicycle over onto its seat and handlebars and were turning the pedals with their hands making the back wheel move furiously fast. As it turned the bigger kids stuck their fingers in the spokes, making a whirring noise.

The secret, of course, was to keep the fingers pointed in the direction in which the wheel was turning. And they were having a jolly ole time. Until. Ronald stuck his finger in there. Until. Ronald's forefinger got caught in the spokes of the wheel. Until. Ronald started screaming bloody murder as he pulled his finger back. To the kids it looked like it was hanging on his hand by a razor-thin strip of skin. They were terror-stricken.

Annie Catherine was in the house, luckily, and she managed to get word to dad at the sawmill in Whitlock. He was home in minutes, it seemed, and picked up the hysterical Ronald, put him in the car and drove him to the doctor. Ronald came home with his hand wrapped in a big bandage halfway up to his elbow. And later dad gave the other kids what-for for letting the baby get that close to the bicycle.

There is one discrepancy in the Kid's remembering; he seems to be the only one in the family who was there. Jacky said he didn't remember it. Ronald said he didn't remember and, besides that, says, "seems to me like there'd be a scar somewhere on one of my hands and there isn't." Still, to this day, the Kid won't say uncle or calf rope. Yo momma.

Poverty drove Peggy and Ronald away from the family. Grandmother decided the log house was no decent place for Peggy to live, so she somehow convinced dad to let Peggy come to Paris to live with her and granddaddy. She must have taken the bike with her because the Kid didn't remember seeing it again around the log house.

Cecil Hopkins, grandmother's brother Willie's boy, took a shine to Ronald and decided that the log house was no place for a baby. He took Ronald home with him where he lived with Aunt Mona. For some reason, though, not long afterward Ronald went to live with grandmother and became her all-time favorite of the Moody kids. "The only one amongst you that ever had a lick of sense was little Ronald. Ronald was the sweetest thang I've ever seen. I guess the only thang that saved him was that he was too young for his daddy's worthlessness to be rubbed off on him. Then that Pearl had to take him. I could kill her for that."

The Kid and Jacky had what probably amounted to the most fun of their childhood there. With dad preoccupied with feeling sorry for himself, drinking and getting the wherewithal to drink some more, there wasn't a whole lot of stiff discipline rampant around the house.

The two boys had the run of the place. And spent weeks exploring every nook and cranny of every building and ditch and woods within walking distance. There was an adventure at every turn of every day. Going out into the woods to pick up wood for the fire was great fun, although sometimes they would forget that the purpose of their mission was to bring home some wood.

Distractions ran rampant: animals, birds, running knee-deep through dry leaves. They took their Roy Rogers (Kid) and Gene Autry (Jacky) cap-guns with them to protect themselves and to shoot themselves out of trouble until dad put a stop to that after he noticed some kind of correlation between the amounts of wood for the fire brought back by the boys and their possession of firearms.

There was no television in the house. None of the remaining Moody's had ever seen a television program. There was no radio in the house. There was horseplay aplenty between the brothers and dad when he was feeling frisky. On particularly delightful nights, dad would pick his old guitar up, sit on a straight-backed chair in front of the blazing fire in the fireplace, rear back and sing to Annie Catherine and the boys for what seemed like hours.

> *"When I was number one*
> *I was always on the run*
> *roll me over in the clover*
> *lay me down*
> *When I was number two*
> *my true love I pursued*
> *roll me over in the clover*
> *lay me down*
> *Roll me ooover in the cloooover*
> *roooooollll me over*
> *lay me doooowwwwn*
> *and doooo it again."*

When he lived somewhere else with people who didn't sing the songs dad liked to sing and the Kid sang the "lay-me-down" song, he got knocked on his ass for singing such a dirty song.

They discovered a couple of worn out tires out back. Those boys rolled those tires hour after hour every day. Up hills. Down hills. Cross country. Stand it up. Give it a shove with your hand. Push it faster and faster alongside it until it runs away from you.

And Snowball loved it. Somebody—the Kid couldn't remember who—had given them Snowball when he was a puppy. Not long after they'd moved to the log house. He'd been a constant friend and playmate to the Kid and Jacky ever since. Snowball was a running fool.

Jacky would hold the tire up while the Kid, who was the smaller of the two, would sit crunched up in the hole. Jacky would then roll the tire down the hill by the house. What a ride! Rolling over and over and over as the tire rolled faster and faster and faster as it bounced down the hill. It felt like. Like. Like bouncing around inside a tire going lickety-split down a bumpy hill. Breathtaking!

Later the closest thrill the Kid could find to riding inside a tire was a rollercoaster which wasn't even in the running for having as much fun. Because he was two years bigger and hard as hell for the Kid to push, Jacky only got about one in five rides but he was a good sport about it.

Saturday was the Kid's and Jacky's favorite day during those months at the log house. When dad had some cash on him. Enough to finance a car trip to the Princess Theatre and some left over for two bags of popcorn. Then leave them alone, because they were in their glory.

Roy Rogers and Trigger rode through that theatre a zillion trillion million times chasing the crooks. Roy always got his man and always won his fight and always came out on top. A real American hero. Man, could he fight! Don't mess with Roy Rogers. Don't even think you can get away with any of that shit. Good is right and right is might and might wins the day and the way. Still, the Kid never figured out how Roy could roll over those campfires as he wrestled freedom from yet another crook and never got burnt.

The two boys would stay in the Princess until someone came in to get them. All day. They'd often see the main feature two or three times. And the serials. Captain Marvel was everything to the brothers that Superman would be to later fanatics. And he was always serialized. One story would last eight or ten weeks, one installment per week. To keep them coming back to see what happened when, say, a car flew off the cliff carrying an innocent family, a diversion forcing Captain Marvel to interrupt his pursuit of the bad guys. And the Kid and Jacky went back every chance they had. They'd spend the next week acting out the more exciting scenes of the previous Saturday's movie. That winter Santa Claus musta known they were stone cowboys and brought them each cap pistols and holsters.

That old DeSoto provided a lot of adventure during the year of the log house. Like the time a tire went flat and dad didn't have a jack so he drove it, with all the kids and Annie Catherine in it, to Puryear, with a flat tire which the gravel road quickly shredded down to a bare wheel.

Some weekends, when times were flush, dad and Annie Catherine would put a little gas and a lotta beer in the back of the DeSoto and take off for the lake. Kentucky Lake. Where the boys would jump in and not come out until somebody came with a warrant. They'd swim under water with their eyes wide open, exploring as far and as deep as they could until their lungs felt like they would explode inside them. Those boys shoulda been ducks.

Dad would come in once in awhile to toss them around and play. Annie Catherine never did go in though. Annie Catherine was kinda standoffish in some ways. She wudn't about to do whatever it was she didn't want to do. It drew the Kid to her like a magnet. He wanted her to be his momma. Sittin' there in her slacks and sleeveless blouse. But, for the Kid for the rest of his life, nobody, not even Annie Catherine, would ever be the momma he was looking for.

Some Sundays dad used to take what was left of the family over to a colored family's house way back up in the woods on a hill. On the backside of nowhere. The Kid now thinks, among the things the location hid, was a still, from whose lead pipes dripped white-lightning which drew dad like a magnet. Back then he thought they went over for a picnic every week or so. There always was one or two possums or coons being fattened up under an overturned sweet potato crate. The Kids knew they'd have some of that meat before they went home that night. And cornbread. And hominy. And greens. Goodies.

The Kid and Jacky had, by then, learned to appreciate even food that was good for them. They liked it all. Except beet pickles which they had made themselves sick on when they stole a quart from the Watsons and ran outside to the end of the back porch and gulped down in five minutes while dad was waiting around front to take them home. And puked themselves sick. Fifty years later and the Kid still turns pale at the sight or smell of beet pickles.

In young lives dotted with special experiences, those Sunday outings were special to the Moody kids.

There were always a bunch of kids waiting to run and play. There were always new places to explore, new treasures to uncover and new thrills to be had. As long as the adults were besotting themselves with whatever it was they besotted themselves with nobody interfered with the business at hand. The business of living a child's life fully.

After one of those Sunday afternoons, they all piled into the DeSoto — the boy's bellies full of barbequed possum and sweet tater, dad and Annie Catherine's bellies full of hooch — and started down the hill toward home. There was a sharp turn at the bottom of the steep hill on which the house sat in the deep Tennessee woods. The brakes went on vacation. The DeSoto didn't negotiate — never even offered a compromise to — the curve but did slam-dunk head on into a medium sized tree at the foot of the hill.

Crash!

The Kid's head felt like somebody had split it in half! Damn! That hurt. A lot.

Annie Catherine was driving as she was wont to do when she figured dad had overfilled his tank. As his forehead hammered the back of the driver's seat, the Kid saw her head bounce off the steering wheel. Annie Catherine yelled. Somebody started to cry. The folks in the house came running down to help.

Dad got out of the car cussing. Dad fiddled with the brakes, had somebody help push the fender out to where it wouldn't rub against the tire and to push the car back onto the grass and dirt road. And away they went again! Mayhaps to sleep. Or steal some chickens. Or find some beer. To further high adventure.

Once in awhile, Sunday would find dad worrying about some of his kids not being with him. And the drunker he got the more he worried. Until finally he'd pile Annie Catherine, Jacky and the Kid in the car and roar down the road to grandmother's house. He'd pull up on the side of the gravel road in front of grandmother's house, lean over Annie Catherine and yell, "I come to see my kids. You stole my kids and I come to take 'em home!"

He'd rant until he ran out of breath, scaring the bejeezus out of Peggy. Ronald was probably too young to let it bother him. He'd keep it up until granddaddy and whichever one of the boys was visiting that day would come out to the car and try to calm him down. And usually he was inconsolable and would try to start a fight with anyone whom he perceived to be interfering with his parental rights. There would be a terrible emotional scene in the front yard. Inevitably. The scenario became so predictable it could have been scripted.

Finally grandmother swore out a peace warrant on dad to keep him away from Peggy because she was so afraid of him. I suspect that fear was the result of dad's drunken behavior and grandmother's continual denunciation of him to anyone who would listen.

The peace bond worked for awhile. Until the combination of moroseness and drunkenness gave him enough courage to flip the bird to everybody in order to see his kids again. Then the big jokester in the sky would hit the reply button and watch, with a grin, as the same old scene played itself out all over again. The pain clearly was too much for either father or kids to bear and far too much to go away.

"Connie Moody don't give a goddamn if you call the law. Connie Moody ain't scared of the law. Ain't no law gonna make me stay away from my kids. You hear me? You hear me, Nell Sutton!"

But somehow he almost always heeded them and allowed himself to be led back to the car where Annie Catherine and the boys waited. Sometimes one of grand-mother's kids would persuade dad to bring Jacky and the Kid out for a week or so visit. Everybody's hearts in their mouths. Peggy visibly crying and nearly hysterical with fear when she gathered enough courage to stick her head through the door.

And they'd take off again to some other place that specialized in dissipating heartbreak. Some beer joint on the flipside of town where Hank Williams and Hank Thompson poured out their beer-drinking, blues-riddled souls six for a quarter. While the guy Sam Garrett left wifeless and drifting sat on a barstool, his elbows form-ing an A-frame to support his head on the bar while one hand fed him a cigarette and the other a Stag beer.

In uniform, of course: a ribbed T-shirt with a pocket over his left breast for his cigarettes. He did not easily melt into the crowd with his receding hairline and his pouty lips and snorty way of talking in that Tennessee drawl.

He was not easily ignored. He'd sit there drinking and smoking and listening until somebody rattled his cage. And after a half dozen beers it didn't take a whole lot to get him going. Then he'd rise up like a bull driven crazy by a red flag. "My name is Connie Moody and by god ain't nobody gonna tell me what to do. And if they try I'll kill 'em. Don't nobody mess with Connie Moody!"

Dad was pissed off at just about everything in the world, especially when he was drunk. And violent. Ended up in a knife fight somewhere over Annie Catherine where he got his lifelong souvenir: a slash that cut the right side of his lip open so bad that his lips weren't aligned properly for rehealing causing dad to have a kind of permanent smirk. Which fit his attitude, come to think of it.

Connie Moody lived more than half of his life suffering the hell of the damned. Of that much he was acutely aware. Every day.

After awhile subsistence living and substantive drinking became a way of life for the Moodys. Not only did he not have worldly wealth, dad was chasing away friends by constantly asking them to babysit the kids and then by compounding the crime by showing up at their house drunk.

It wasn't too long before the combination of his assoholism and the shame of allowing himself to be swept down into the pit of self-pity and loathing drove dad away from almost all. What had once been symbiotic relations became totally one-sided. All favors for dad; no favors from dad. All money loaned to dad; no repayment from dad. All promises from dad; no promises kept by dad. He sponged off those who had and then lowered his sights to those who didn't.

The neighbors. The only people he could ask to keep us overnight were the colored family up the road. People who had as little as Connie Moody had through no fault of their own. Who worked in the massuh's fields every day all day long to scratch out a bare existence which Connie Moody asked them to share with his kids so he could take Annie Catherine out honky-tonking.

He'd pull the DeSoto up in front of the little wooden shack a mile up the road from the log house, roll down the driver's side window and yell out, "How y'all!" The introduction to imposing the kids on those poor people another night. Rough wood floors. Rough construction. Yard worn bare by kids playing and chickens scratching.

But the Kid and Jacky didn't see any of that. What they saw was a place where they were welcome. Where there was food and a warm bed. Until one night the Kid heard the man, speaking very softly, complain to his wife about "puttin' up with them white folks stuff," and, "it's a shame what he doin' to them kids. He oughter be 'shamed."

Not until years later did he realize how great the sacrifice must have been. The enforced sharing of what little they had, which was barely enough for themselves, with those white kids down the road. And it was reinforced. A person of color in Tennessee in nineteen-forty-nine dare not say no to a white person's request. Not if they didn't want to risk their health and their lives. While it was true there was bonhomie and kindness and sharing that was genuine, it was also true that they had no real choice, no matter how friendly Connie Moody tried to make the whole thing out to be.

One night while dad was leaning against the car talking to a man, Annie Catherine opened her purse and came up with a half pint of apricot brandy. "Here, Kid, have a taste," she urged as she pressed the open mouth of the bottle to his lips. It burned like fire, then tasted like strong-flavored peaches.

He loved it because Catherine had given it to him. He loved anything Catherine gave to him. He didn't even mind walking around with his head awhirl for awhile after they'd taken off for their bar of the night.

On the rare occasions when dad was too embarrassed to drop the two boys off at the neighbors' house they'd take them to the beer gardens with them. The boys would spend the night being entertained by increasingly drunk patrons who tousled their hair, murmured shit about "poor little orphans", and pressed pennies and nickels, even an occasional dime, into their palms. The youngsters mostly drank cold drinks and rarely had a hangover the next day.

One night at a bar dad and Annie Catherine got into one of their pitched verbal battles replete with insults, threats, and appeals for heavenly retribution. Sobriety was not a preapproved requisite of the discussion. They were both drunk as skunks. Even the boys knew that from the slurring and the slobbering and the slopping and the slumping. "Come on, Jacky, we're leaving. You too, Kid."

"The Kid can stay with me if he wants to."

The Kid nods yes. Vigorously.

Dad and Jacky stalked out and drove away in the DeSoto, leaving Annie Catherine and the Kid behind.

"They'll be back, your daddy's jest tryin' to scare me some," she said.

When they had not returned and closing time came around, she started looking for a ride home for the two of them. Which wasn't hard. Seemed like every man in there liked her just as much as the Kid did. Which was a lot. Finally one of them said okay.

In the car Annie Catherine said, "No, there won't be any of that and there won't be any of that even if the boy wasn't in the car. I'm with Connie and until he and I split I'm with him. I don't wanna hurt your feelings, but that's just the way it is."

The front door was locked.

They finally roused Jacky who let them in. As they were standing in the tiny hallway between the boys' bedroom and the living room/master bedroom, he fearfully announced, "You better watch out Catherine. Dad put a hammer under his pillow to get you when you came home."

Annie Catherine quietly opened the door to where her husband was snoring loudly. She tiptoed into the room, over to the bed, reached gently under the pillow dad was sleeping on and pulled out a ball-peen hammer, and walked out into the hallway. "He was gonna kill me, the son-of-a-bitch was really gonna kill me! I'll just hide this where he won't never find it, leastways not anytime soon."

Both the Kid and Jacky were sure dad was going to kill her when he woke up. Instead he sat on the edge of the bed, rubbed his head and acted as though nothing untoward had happened the previous night. Nothing.

Ding Dong the Dog is Gone

Somewhere in a soggy park in a dirty city on a rainy day in Indiana in nineteen-forty-nine dad walked back to the car alone. "Where's Snowball?" The Kid asked. "Damn dog ran away," dad answered in that snorty kinda way he talked sometimes, like he was trying to talk and blow his nose at the same time. "I took him over there by some bushes so he could do his business and the damn dog took off. He's gone. Long gone. That dog ain't coming back. So we might as well get on with it."

Jacky and the Kid were near tears. "Can't we wait for him? He'll be here in a minute, Dad. I know he will!"

"Well just for a minute. You know we can't wait very long. We've got a long trip ahead of us still."

Two minutes later dad climbed into the old burgundy DeSoto coupe, cranked it up and drove on up the road toward Detroit. With a few stops along the way. Within twenty minutes the DeSoto was parked outside a ramshackle wooden building weatherproofed with beer signs. "Play pinball," he said. "I'll make us some money for the trip."

Jacky and the Kid lay on the stuff piled high on the backseat waiting for dad to return, both just below blubbering for the fair and radiant Snowball.

Annie Catherine switched her cigarette from her left hand to the right and reached back to pat their hands. "I don't know about your daddy sometimes," she said. "I've lived with him nearly two years and I haven't figured him out yet."

"Snowball didn't run away, did he, Catherine?"

"No Kid, to tell you the truth, I don't think so. I think your daddy dropped him somewhere because he doodooed in the backseat. That's what I think. But I also think there's a chance he'll find a good home and somebody who'll love him just as much as you and Jacky do. I'm sorry, but there's nothing I can do about it. Not when Connie Moody's got his mind made up."

"We shoulda left him at home, shouldn't we?"

"You can't worry about it now, boys. It's too late and it won't do any good."

It took longer than that summer to forgive dad for dropping off Snowball in a park somewhere in Indiana on the way to Detroit where dad didn't get a job anyway.

What the Kid remembered mostly was that dad had lied. First he told them they could take Snowball to Detroit. And then he did something to Snowball. And then he lied about it. The Kid knew exactly what had happened. Dad got tired of messing with the dog and of the dog messing in the car because dad wouldn't stop and let the dog go to the bathroom. So dad got rid of the dog with the white hair and curly tail.

He shouldn't have lied about it. He should have known kids know when grownups lie about things that are important to them.

...

Several times that summer dad and Catherine dragged the Kid away from the spinning tires of the world's most perfect playground to drive him up to the Henry County Health Department for his pre-school shots. The first time was fun. Driving through the tree-lined streets up to a big brick building. Going inside.

Until some asshole poked a needle the size of a hayrake into his arm creating lasting pain and, surely, permanent damage that'd prevent the Kid from ever-more using his arm for anything more strenuous than slinging in a sling. The summer of nineteen-forty-nine marked the beginning of the Kid's lifelong aversion to hypodermic needles.

...

Puryear School. First grade. Miss Pillow. Tall. Grey hair found in a tightly twisted braid around her small head. Skinny. Gaunt eyes that only turned merry when you got close enough for a good look. In real life Miss Pillow was a good, caring teacher. Except the Kid would wonder later on how come he hadn't memorized the alphabet by the time he and Jacky skipped school and town for other beds and breakfasts.

...

Getting Up the Hard Way

In forty-nine Aunt Louise kept saying, "You kids need to get away from that house. I don't care if he is my brother, you don't need to be there and see what you're seeing and have to take it. You don't have enough to eat. You dress like little tramps. There's nobody that looks after you. You'd be better off where Peggy and Ronald are. Anywhere away from your daddy. Now I'm not saying your daddy don't love you; I'm sure as I can be that he does, but he can't take care of hisself, much less you kids."

Jacky and the Kid used to visit Aunt Louise a lot, especially when there was no food in the house or when dad and Annie Catherine were planning a protracted booze party. Aunt Louise was always going on like that. She was dad's only sister and was the Kid's mom's best friend until mom got killed by that goddamn drunkard Sam Garrett.

This time the Kid apparently listened because it was getting so bad he and Jacky were being locked out of the house most days and had to wait around in the cold, often for hours, before those two showed up.

One afternoon, they took the school bus home to the airy log house on Whitlock Road and, sure enough, the door was locked. Again. No one was home. Again. The Kid took Jacky's hand and said, "Let's go, Jacky. Like Aunt Louise said."

Jacky, who was two years older, hesitated. He loved his father more than anyone else in the world. Even then the Kid was partial to women; he loved his step-mom, Annie Catherine, best, but not enough to stop him from trying to find some food and warmth and constancy. Unless Annie Catherine came by and gave him a snort of peach brandy and a hug, then he would have followed her anywhere.

The Kid tugged on his brother's hand. Jacky started crying. The Kid didn't feel so well hisself, but continued to feel the push to leave, to get out of there and to do it quickly before the folks got home. There was no question, running away would not have happened if Connie and Catherine had just *been there*.

They walked down the gravel road to their next door neighbor's house, probably not much further than a long city block, and knocked on the door. The neighbors welcomed the boys, fed them supper and listened to their story about what Aunt Louise had said and about coming home most nights to a dark, locked house with no way in until the drunks got home.

The neighbors clucked sympathetically as the pair filled up their bellies with cornbread and beans and warmed up their bodies inside the cozily heated house.

The neighbor man drove them to the Washatorium in Puryear where he telephoned Aunt Louise. Aunt Louise and Uncle Nolan drove to Puryear, picked up Jacky and the Kid and drove them the eight miles to Paris where grandmother lived.

Grandmother's inn was all full up and what the hell were they going to do with the Kid and Jacky? Certainly they couldn't send them back to their good for nuthin' trifling daddy.

She called for Uncle J and Uncle Sam to come and see what could be done. Uncle J took Jacky; Uncle Sam took the Kid and put them in their respective pickup trucks and hauled them out to their respective farms near Mansfield.

Jacky lasted a few months. He didn't like them; they didn't like him. He wound up at grandmother's house where he stayed until the infamous sweet potato-and-butter-smashed-against-the-refrigerator incident.

The Kid wasn't so lucky. As the tale unfolded years later, he learned that Connie, the Kid's daddy, had had an affair of sorts with Aunt Naomi, Uncle Sam's wife. It seems Uncle Sam had discovered this copulative adventure and had not been overjoyed nor even mildly pleased. In fact, some say, Uncle Sam was so pissed off he could chew nails, but he settled for hating Connie Moody and all of Connie Moody's bloodline until the planet Earth was destroyed by the fire of the second-coming.

That's the setting the Kid entered in nineteen-forty-nine. A foster home headed by an ill-tempered sumbitch who hated his father's guts and who would take it out on the son of the accused for as long as he was bigger than the Kid so that he could manhandle him at will until his psyche was scarred forever more.

The farm was just about the most beautiful sight the Kid had ever seen. Plenty of room to run and play. Woods to explore. And a playmate to take Jacky's place. Cousin Joel was only a year younger. Young as he was he felt like he was breathing in a wonderful life when he saw the house sitting there on the gentle slope of hill, its clapboard a mixture of green and white.

The farm sloped downward to the railroad track. The road ran smack dab into the house. Beyond the house in the yard was the outdoor two-seater toilet which they used all year long, including the times when your butt just about froze to the hole; the smokehouse where the home-cured hams and bacon hung under their protective coating of scum; the chicken house where the eggs got laid for human folk and egg-sucking dogs and egg-swallowing snakes; and Aunt Naomi's garden right behind that.

Farther on down the hill was the pigpen with Rosie and her friends. Rosie, the big fat sow, had it in for the Kid. One day, at Uncle Sam's behest, the Kid had jumped into a stall in the barn to drive Rosie into the pigpen. He clapped his hands, waved his arms and shooed her out of the stall. Except instead of going like a good little fat sow, she turned on him and let him know she wasn't about to be pushed around by some snot-nosed skinny kid. Instead of meekly going, she grunted that savage grunt of hers, backed up to the far side of the stall and took her last stand. That scared the Kid.

Then, brazened by his fear, she charged the Kid who damn near pissed his pants as he scooted up the side of the edge of a two-by-six and where he would have happily stayed for the rest of his life had not Uncle Sam rushed back to make him do it again until he got it right, which he never could and which may have been about the only time Uncle Sam had to wind up doing the Kid's job. Even Uncle Sam could see the Kid was real close to being scared to death. And let him off with a few salty words of reprimand. No blood. One in a row.

Rosie, who was so sweet to the rest of them, never let the Kid forget she'd eat his ass for breakfast if she ever got close enough. He believed her.

He never did get close enough although he still had to help slop the hogs every day. Aunt Naomi kept a five gallon bucket in the kitchen which she filled with every scrap of food the family didn't eat like potato peels, eggshells, anything that she thought could be digested by Rosie and the clan, including dirty dishwater.

Once a day, the Kid would put a scoop of bran, for added nutrition, into the bucket, stir it up with a long wooden paddle and take it down to the pigpen and pour it into the pig trough and watch them porkers make fools of themselves as they rushed and grunted and pulled and nipped and jockeyed about for best feeding position.

I think they wouldn't have been so eager if they'd known they would be brought, one by one, one January or February morning, shot in the middle of the forehead with a twenty-two caliber rifle, strung up, cut open, and winding up on the kitchen table to be eaten. As noble as it was — keeping us all alive for another year — I suspect those porkers would have been less eager to belly up to the trough.

To the right of the pigpen — the Kid didn't learn until later that a pigpen is formally a sty — was the barnyard. The barnyard was mostly hard-packed dirt splotched with cow shit and mule turds. Except when it was raining. Then the barnyard was an awful smelling ankle-deep mixture that you had to muck through to feed the cows and mules and hogs. The mule turds don't smell that bad. I think it has something to do with the fact that mules are sexless creatures who have involuntarily swapped semen for sweat.

Sitting in the middle of the barnyard was the corncrib, life-giver to all the domesticated beasties who provided sustenance for Uncle Sam and Aunt Naomi and Joel Sutton. And later, even little Linda. The Kid wasn't sure then, or now, whether he was one of the folks who

71

belonged in the farmhouse or one of the beasties who belonged in the barn or pasture or pigpen or henhouse. He'd been brought in—reluctantly, he'd heard—in answer to a direct appeal from grandmother to Uncle Sam because nobody else wanted him except maybe his dad who couldn't hack fatherhood and mainline alcohol at the same time.

There was always someone there; he didn't come home after school to find the doors locked and nobody home. It felt good to do chores around the house. Carrying water in a half-gallon Mason jar to Uncle Sam working with the mules in the cotton patch or cultivating corn with the tractor. Fetching the cows at night for milking. Hoeing cotton and Aunt Naomi's garden. Feeding the animals. Learning to milk the cows, which he never got very good at.

Even the hard work in the fields when he was six and seven. During the cotton harvest in the fall of nineteen-fifty, when he was seven years old, the Kid picked one hundred pounds of cotton in a single day, and hasn't ever been any prouder of anything in his life.

He also helped with corn planting and haying and the making of sorghum molasses—Uncle Sam had built a mule-powered sorghum mill just beyond the front yard. The sorghum stalks, which looked a lot like cornstalks, were thrown into the hopper and crushed and drained of their juice by a grindstone driven by a mule walking slowly in circles all day for days on end.

Uncle Sam didn't know a whole lot about farming. But he tried. Sometimes. He took a lot of Agriculture Extension Service courses to learn the intricacies. And while he was attending classes, which were held ten miles down the road in Paris, he'd take Aunt Naomi, Joel and the Kid to visit with neighbors. Mostly they'd just talk. The drone of their voices was like a lullaby.

It was all heaven.

Until.

The vengeful uncle put on his executioner's mask, took up whips and belts and tree limbs and threats of eternal damnation, knocked on the door of the homey house, came in and went to work.

With a will.

Uncle Sam beat him with a belt until his legs bled because he had failed to memorize his ABC's as instructed within the time allowed. And couldn't because he was six and couldn't read cursive writing which is how Uncle Sam had written the alphabet.

"The pencil you brought home from school is not the one I gave you this morning. Where did you steal this? Get me a switch from that tree, Kid. Don't you dare run away from me. I'll show you who's boss. I knew it wouldn't work out. You just got too much daddy in you. You ain't never gonna be any good. Now, where did you get that pencil?"

He held the Kid's left hand in the air with his own left hand as he flailed the wood against the Kid's dancing flesh with the other.

"I don't know, Uncle Sam. I don't know." Terrified. Hopping. Looking for escape from the fire of the lashing. On tiptoes. Dancing to the devil's tune Uncle Sam played on his six year old flesh. Unendurable pain from the sting of the switch raining down relentlessly on his buttocks and legs.

"Where'd you get that pencil, Kid? This is for your own good. You are not going to be a thief. I won't let you. Where did you get that pencil? Where did you steal it? Tell me. You'd better tell me, Kid, or you won't be able to walk for a week. Do you understand me?"

"I don't know!" Hysterically.

"Doesn't this hurt enough? You better tell me. I don't know why I waste my time, you'll never be any better than that daddy of yours. But I won't let you get away with this. Where did you steal that pencil!"

"I found it! I found it! I found it on the playground! I'm sorry! I'm sorry!" The Kid sobbed and sobbed and sobbed, not knowing what to say once the truth had been dismissed.

The beating stopped only when Uncle Sam's arms got too tired to slash the Kid's bleeding flesh any further.

And so it went. For months.

Sheer joy for the Kid when he could switch to his bird mode: soaring high in the sky, free as the hawks and buzzards that blazed about looking for lunch and dinner - and napping peacefully on the wing.

Pure terror when Uncle Sam decided he had sinned.

Since Uncle Sam was one of grandmother's very favorites, she readily—and frequently—excused his harsh behavior, blaming it on the war. "Sam Sutton was the nicest, quietest kid you've ever seen," she'd say. "Until he went overseas. He saw too much for a kid that age. And did too much. His best friend in the Army was killed in the same foxhole where Sam was. I'm not making excuses for Sam, but I do know he wouldn't be like this if it hadn't been for the war."

Uncle Sam had gone into the infantry during World War II when he was seventeen or eighteen. His division was the one whose logo was the skull of a cow which decorated several dishes in Grandmother's house. After basic training he was shipped to Italy where, as they say, he "engaged" the enemy. And apparently learned how to beat the hell out of people who were a lot smaller and weaker than he.

The Kid got beaten when he screwed up. The Kid got beaten when Joel screwed up and the Kid got blamed. The Kid got beaten when he showed someone at school welts on his back and legs.

Manners. One morning after breakfast, the Kid, who had mannerly kept his left hand under the table while he ate with his right, who had chewed with his mouth closed, and who thought he'd done okay, was walking from the living room onto the front porch when Uncle Sam smacked his cheek with his open hand nearly knocking the Kid off his feet. "Do you know why you got that?"

"No sir."

"Two reasons. One: you took the last of the eggs; you know you're not supposed to do that. You know you're supposed to always leave some in the bowl for other people. And two: you scraped the eggs out of the bowl. Don't you have any manners, boy? You know you're supposed to pick them up with the spoon and lift them from the bowl to your plate."

The Kid was a six, and later seven, year old emotional basket case.

He was also a bedwetter. He couldn't count the times he was awakened by something warm seeping down his legs and up to his waist. Befuddled. Until he was suddenly aware of what it was, where it was coming from and, worst of all, whom it was coming from. And he'd quake; wish the wetness away, wishing the accident away, and wishing he could somehow do something to make it never to have occurred. And he could hardly breathe from the terror of discovery. And he knew Aunt Naomi would find out and tell Uncle Sam and get the belt for it. Again. And again. And again.

There aren't a lot of happy mornings for bedwetters who know they're facing ninety-nine to life every time they piss themselves in their sleep. And it didn't help his self-confidence a whole lot for Uncle Sam and Aunt Naomi to talk about his incontinence in loud voices with his uncles and aunts at grandmother's house. Voices loud enough for other kids to hear. Kids who would tease him mercilessly. "You wet the bed! You wet the bed! You wet the bed! You oughta hang your head!"

He'd wake up in the middle of the night with the urge to pee and be afraid to make noise and wake up Uncle Sam and Aunt Naomi, so he'd lie there until his bladder pushed him up to standing, then he'd jiggle his body to drive the urge away. It seemed like it would never stop. There was no slop jar in the room he shared with Joel for middle of the night peetime.

Scared half to death, he sometimes would pee on the wood floor around the edge of the linoleum rug so he wouldn't disturb anyone. Then, of course, he'd be discovered and promised that his was a criminal career close to full-bloom and that pretty soon his name would be in the newspaper right there alongside the names of all those other murderers and thieves and troublemakers.

Once the Kid shit his pants in the morning as he walked to the bus stop a half mile from the house. He didn't know why. He never knew why. But he never forgot that awful smell he had to live with all day, including both ways on the bus and in front of Dovey Cole whom he adored.

School was wonderful. Especially when his overalls were shit-free. There were people there who actually liked him and treated him like they liked him and he was dying to go home with every one of them that ever did anything nice.

And church. Oh, Lordy, was there ever a community in the state of Tennessee that wasn't foolish about going to church? Every Sunday they'd go to Mansfield Baptist Church: Sunday School at ten o'clock, preaching at eleven o'clock, Training Union at six o'clock, preaching at seven o'clock, prayer meeting Wednesday night. Every Sunday and every Wednesday. A small church, but proud, they would have said. Brother Presson up there talking about salvation and Jesus and heaven and how wonderful life after life would be. One of the few Southern Baptist ministers the Kid would ever see not screaming and ranting and foaming at the mouth.

And the inevitable bean salad for dinner after church.

Once in awhile Uncle Sam would drive the Dodge into Paris for drinks and a good time. Of course, there was always a credible reason for going; pick up some parts or feed or consult with the Agricultural Extension agent. Aunt Naomi often sent Joel and the Kid along, not so much to get them out of her hair, I think, as to keep him from stopping at the beer joint for a six pack. If that was her intention it didn't always work. When Uncle Sam had a big thirst he was gonna quench it.

He actually was a gentler person when he was smashed than when he was stone-cold sober, wielding that skin-slashing belt buckle against his least favorite nephew's nearest flesh.

Like the time he stopped at a beer garden and had a couple or more. Came out, drove to a toy store and bought each of the boys a small wooden train. When he came back to the truck and handed them over, you'd a thought it was Christmas. And it had its desired effect. The boys didn't care what he did after that, their attention had the trains to keep them busy.

Sometime in the afternoon he brought out a couple of empty ice cream containers like those you see in Baskin Robbins — round with strips of metal on the top and bottom. Apparently, that was Aunt Naomi's surprise. He brought them out, put them on the floorboard, and told the boys to "watch these" and returned his attention to the more important agenda of the day. And they watched them. They did. For at least an hour or two.

Until the Kid got the idea that those metal rings would be perfect train tracks. Of course they had to be taken off first and that might ruin Aunt Naomi's ice cream containers. But probably not. They should be alright without the reinforcers. Surely.

They weren't alright.

The bottoms fell out.

And they weren't worth a damn as train tracks.

Aunt Naomi was extremely unhappy and wasn't real shy about broadcasting that fact in a loud shrill voice that cut like a buzzsaw through your nerves. Made you jump, then shiver.

Aunt Naomi had softness and looks and womanhood that sometimes appealed to the Kid, but that temper would flare up like a mini-nuclear blast whenever she got fired up. And it didn't have to be world-class to get caught in her craw. One day the Kid opened the kitchen door and stopped, eyes big as saucers, to see her taking a sponge bath, naked down to her blue panties. Damn! By the time he realized what he was looking at Aunt Naomi had thrown a bar of soap and washrag at him, propelled by a screeching demand for him to get the hell out, right now!

They didn't have a bathroom on the inside of the house. They hauled their water from a well in the backyard and later from the pumphouse after they'd installed an electric pump to do the hauling for them. For everyday bathing they sponged off. Manually. An aluminum washpan half full of cold water. Soap. And a washcloth — what they nowadays call a facecloth. There wasn't a whole lot of attention placed on hygiene because it wasn't so easy back then to wash your hands every time you peed or pooped. Or so convenient.

Bad as it was, sometimes it wasn't. So much to explore. The Kid would go down to the pasture and watch tumblebugs by the hour as they made dungballs out of cow shit, rolling it up like doughballs with their back legs.

Like when Jacky and he roamed all over the country from the Whitlock Road log house. Rabbits. Squirrels. Birds. Creeks. And, especially, woods which would take a lifetime to explore fully and ferret out all the big and little hiding places and discover all their wonders.

In later years, the Kid would mostly remember the beatings and Uncle Sam railing against everything he did, but there were times when it almost felt like he had a family. Aunt Naomi would usually send him off to school with a country ham on biscuit sandwich, which he would dump as soon as he got out of sight from the house because he then hated country ham.

Thirty years later he would rue all that which he'd thrown to the side of the road.

There were two other houses, not counting the colored families, along the road that ran from Mansfield Road to Uncle Sam's house. But none with school-aged kids, so school officials decided it wasn't worth the expense for the school bus to trek all the way down to pick up the Kid. Which is why he walked. Later he would wonder where the colored kids went to school. Or whether they went at all. He would wonder how they got to class. If they had them. Or if anyone gave a rats ass.

He loved Joel like a brother and still remembers him as much closer than a cousin. Among the holes of pain and chastisement and bitterness, there was a palliation born of the resilience of childhood and the comradeship he shared with Joel. They were constant friends, even when the Kid got blamed for whatever crimes Joel had committed — because the Kid *had* to be at fault.

The Kid's head rattled as he stood in the cornfield on a late November's day. Dusk was growing. He had been pulling corn from their stalks and tossing the ears into the mule driven wagon all day. He was dead-dog tired. His head hurt. His arms were sore. His legs were sore. But he knew he was at Uncle Sam's mercy. No rest until Uncle Sam said there was rest. Joel had gone to the house hours ago, although Aunt Naomi was still out there. She'd come out to help after dinner at noontime.

Grab.

Pull.

Toss in the wagon.

Grab.

Pull.

Toss.

Until he felt like a robot.

But winter would soon be here and the corn had to be in the crib — all of it — before the fields got too wet from winter rain. Even farm wagons can't haul themselves full of corn through knee-deep mud.

So they worked.

Only the mules and Uncle Sam never seemed to tire. Uncle Sam never paused his harangue to keep up and do it right and to go faster — addressed to the Kid, of course. If he'd talked to Aunt Naomi like that she'd neuter him right then and there.

When it was too dark to see all the ears of corn, Uncle Sam, the twentieth century double of Simon LaGree, called it quits. Aunt Naomi went to the house to fix supper. Uncle Sam and the Kid took the mules to the barn where they unhitched them and led them to their stalls and banquets of corn and hay. Then milked the cows. And slopped the hogs. And the Kid got the eggs from the hen house lest they be stolen by egg-sucking dogs or snakes during the night.

Finally, supper was over and the Kid and Joel went to bed in the front room that also doubled as a living room. By the time the Kid's head hit the pillow he was fast asleep.

The next morning Aunt Naomi called the boys from the kitchen.

"Okay now, kids. It's time to get up and face the day."

"Get up. Get up!"

The Kid woke up first. Scared to death. His side of the bed was soaking wet.

He had peed the bed. Oh, no. Why couldn't he get through just one week where there weren't so many complications to his life? Why? Why? Why?

Another beating. He hoped it would come quickly and be over with.

The good part about having the humungous pain in the back of his skull was that he wouldn't be able to feel much of the beating.

Overpowering.

The Kid put both hands around his neck and pressed against the back of his skull to ease the pain.

It didn't work.

He threw back the covers, trying to be nonchalant while not exposing the urine-soaked sheets, sat on the side of the bed and pulled his bibbed overall legs over his. Then was up like a flash.

And down like a flash.

He crumpled onto the floor like a limp dishrag.

"What's wrong, Kid?" Aunt Naomi wanted to know.

"Nothing," he responded as he pushed himself off the floor. To crumple again.

"I cccan't wwwwalk," he stammered.

"I'll help," she said, as she rose quickly from her chair. And he knew she was seriously concerned because Aunt Naomi was not one to quickly move anywhere unless you were looking at her without any clothes on.

She pulled the Kid into a standing position then relaxed her hold a moment to see if he could stand now. He would have fallen if she hadn't caught him.

"Sam, get in here. Something's wrong with the Kid."

By the time Uncle Sam got there, the Kid could hardly sit. His muscles were deserting him. All at once.

What was it?

They wrapped him in a quilt, dumped him into the Dodge and rushed him to Noble's Hospital in Paris where Doctor Neumann took his temperature, asked a few questions and advised them to rush the Kid to Isolation Hospital in Memphis, one hundred-thirty-two miles away.

"I'm afraid the Kid's got polio," he said.

He was right.

Limp Legs and Santa Claus

The Kid lay in the back seat of the brand new bright green Pontiac. "We gotta get 'im there as fast as we can, Arlan. Doctor said the quicker the better." "I'm doing ninety-five, Sam. Any faster and we just might land upside down in one of those fields out there."

Arlan Stewart was married to Aunt Naomi's sister Hilda. He owned the ESSO gas station in Paris. He also owned a brand new car that would take the Kid to Isolation Hospital in Memphis. Less than an hour ago Doctor Newman had diagnosed the Kid with poliomyelitis. Since he'd gotten out of bed, falling flat on his ass that November morning in nineteen-fifty, paralysis had slowly encompassed most of the rest of the Kid's body. If it reached his lungs before Memphis they'd be toting a corpse to Isolation Hospital.

The Kid was wrapped up in a blanket in the backseat. Arlan was driving, Uncle Sam riding shotgun. Shooting along U.S. 79 like it was greased lightning. Towns whizzing by like meteorites. McKenzie. Milan. Brownsville.

If the two in the front were scared, they shoulda been there lying behind them.

Yesterday the Kid had been standing by the mule-drawn wagon helping to harvest corn in the field. This morning he couldn't stand. Period. Tonight he couldn't move anything that he could think of. Period. Seven years old and all used up. No more running. No more walking. No more bringing the cows in from the pasture of a night. No more playing with Joel. He couldn't move.

The Kid was scared that he was as close to death as he could get without falling over the precipice.

Isolation Hospital welcomes you. All ye who can't walk or crawl or knock the hands of torture away from your frail carcass, welcome.

Isolation Hospital is where new cases of polio from northern Mississippi and west Tennessee stayed until they were no longer contagious. The Shelby County Health Department tossed the new polio people into their specially prepared antiseptic dungeons.

First thing they did to the Kid was take him to a cold green examination room and shove a needle up his spine. "Right in here, Mister Sutton," the nurse said to Uncle Sam who carried the Kid in his arms. "Over on the table. Take his clothes off down to his underpants and I'll put this sheet over him until the doctor comes in." The doctor came in, raised the sheet and began the torture of the spinal tap. "This won't take long, Kid. It'll hurt a little bit but it'll soon be over. It won't be bad. You'll see. Nurse, hand me that needle."

The Kid may as well have been kidnapped by Martians and taken to Planet Eleven for examination by a race of alien beings who got their jollies off by inflicting pain on people from the planet Earth. Of course, you don't have to leave Earth to find them. You could send a spy into an examining room at Isolation Hospital in Memphis, Tennessee, one cold winter's night in November, the Year of Our Lord, nineteen-fifty.

The Kid was shivering from the cold hammering against his naked skin and from the fear pounding ever more fiercely against his chest with each succeeding heartbeat.

"Hold him still. She's going to need some help, Mister Sutton. Will you get over here and hold his legs? Okay, Kid, try to relax. The more you relax the less it's going to hurt. Relax."

"Oooooowwwwww!" That needle must have been as big as a milk bottle as much as it hurt. The Kid wept and wiggled. The more he wiggled, the more tightly the nurse and Uncle Sam held him to keep him still.

"Oooooowwwwww!" The wail of a wild thing sending out a haunting, helpless cry for help, a cry that joined a thousand others just like it deep inside the walls of Isolation Hospital. Where the only company it would find would be others of its own kind, for it would never find comfort in the hollow hearts of the assigned purveyors of caregiving.

"Oooooowwwwww!" The Kid now knew that it would never end, that the doctor's first lie would lay under a half ton of others he'd pile on top of each, promising "not much pain," or "it'll be over soon," or "there that's not so bad, is it?" He would never feel more helpless or more alone than he did that night in Memphis, Tennessee.

Like all good things, though, it passed. Into a hospital room built for two. And some sleep to refresh the pain and fear. By the time the Kid had slipped into a new kind of moonlight madness Uncle Sam and Arlan were long gone, taking the green Pontiac on the home trek. And there wasn't one single human being on the face of that whole corner of southwest Tennessee called Memphis that the Kid knew. Somebody figured out a new definition for abandonment that night.

"Hi, I've got chickenpox." The Kid opened his eyes and started to wipe the sleep from his eyes until he realized with a start that he couldn't move his arms. But he was awake. In a super-sized baby bed with sides like prison bars that could be lifted or lowered by people who could move their arms and hands. "My name's Billy. What's your name?" His head could still turn. He looked over toward the voice and found a scrawny kid sitting on the other bed in the room looking like he'd been splashed by a moving car wheel running over a pool of red paint.

"Hi, I'm Kid," Kid replied. "I can't move my arms."

A black lady dressed in white brought a tray in and sat it on Billy's bed. And went away. And came back with another tray of food she sat on a bedside table for the Kid. "Can you move enough to eat, honey? Okay, I'm gonna have to feed you til you can do it for yourself."

The Kid must have looked stricken. "Don't you worry, sugar, you gonna be alright. Can't nothin' hurt cha as long as I'm here. You hear me? Now take a bite." Oatmeal, toast, and milk. Yum yum.

Somebody else fed the Kid his lunch. Around midafternoon a white lady dressed in white came into the room carrying a tray filled with little glasses of something that looked a lot like tomato juice. And a shot. Seeing the needle near 'bout sent the Kid into seizures. "I don't need a shot. I really don't. I'm feeling a lot better. And I'll be able to move real soon. I think I can move a little right now. Please don't give me a shot. Please." His thumping heart turned on the tears and upped the hysteria. If fright could kill he would have been dead before nurse white could say, "this shot's not even for you. It's for Billy. All I've got for you is some juice."

The next week was Thanksgiving. No visitors. Don't matter who they are, how alone he is, or how far they had to come to see him. Uncle Sam, Aunt Naomi and Joel drove all the way to Memphis to see the Kid. Nurse white pushed his bed to the window so he could see them as they stood in the snow in the parking lot.

Snow?

Yep. There had been a record freeze in west Tennessee the week after the Kid got the "viri" *(the nonstandard, jocular plural of virus – because if there was anything dad wasn't, it was standard -- CL).* Uncle Sam's well pump froze and cost him a pretty penny to repair. Water pipes all over Henry County popped a vein and cost a lot of pretty pennies. Got down to below zero.

The first the Kid ever knew anything about it was when he saw his visitors standing in the snow down in the hospital parking lot. People he'd spent twenty-four hours a day with for a year. And now he could only see them for a minute or two and then through a second floor window as they waved.

Lonesome as Hank Williams' whippoorwill ever was. "Hi!" He couldn't wave. He could look, though. He could look at the snow. Couldn't play in it. Although he wanted to. He couldn't remember the last time he'd seen snow. Maybe never. All he knew was that he should be out there "doing it", even though as he lay in bed "it" was only a feeling, a rush of excitement that filled him up until it got to the place where he had to move to get up and get out and do "it".

In spite of not being able to move any part of his body except his head, the Kid was making friends on the inside lickety-split. Always the schmoozer, the Kid shoulda been a politician. "Hey! What's yer name? I can't move anything except my head. What can you move?"

The art of conversation was born in those weeks when the tongue was the most active sign of life on a body that once had dared jump from the tallest branch of the tree just to show brother Jacky he was braver than him. A body that had saved itself on more than one occasion by escaping from the kids with the butcher knives. A body that had done a lively, if gruesome, dance more than once to the tune of Uncle Sam's singing belt buckle.

And they talked back. A twenty year old girl spent her life in a respirator — which some persisted in calling an "iron lung" in later years — because she couldn't breathe without it. The viri got her lungs, too. All the Kid knew was that she was beautiful and that when he grew up he wanted to marry her. Lying there with her head sticking out of this big cylinder, her hair spread like fine silk on the pillow. Her beautiful eyes looking into his. The Kid was in love again. Move over Linda Lou Hart. Move over Annie Catherine Bray. Move over Dovey Cole.

Days went by slowly in the hospital where there was little to do. There was no television and no radio. These were the days when hospitals were supposed to be quiet and, by god, they were kept quiet. The silence was often, however, the overwhelming sound of boredom.

Until the Kid's viri backed off a bit. One day the Kid accidentally flexed a finger. Yippee! From then on it was like lava flowing uphill, but flowing nonetheless. More fingers moved. Then a wrist. And an elbow. Until both hands worked all the way through the shoulders! Hallelujah!

Now for the comic books which rained down on Isolation Hospital like manna. Seems like everybody figured young kids penned up in isolation away from their families and friends could use some good literature of the kind that came prepackaged in line drawings on squares printed on cheap paper and covered with slick paper with big drawings.

The Kid devoured comic books with the same fervor that would power him most of his life through love and hobbies and habits of all like.

Just in time for Christmas vacation. There was some soul in someone in Isolation Hospital 'cuz they let Uncle Sam take the Kid home to Henry County for a few days over Christmas. He borrowed somebody's car and packed him in blankets on the backseat and set off.

Once Uncle Sam had to stop and lift the Kid out of the car so he could pee on the side of the road. Which was a trick since the Kid couldn't stand and Uncle Sam only had two arms and hands with which to hold the Kid and help him pee at the same time. But what's a little urine among kinfolk. Right?

Aunt Naomi and Joel were standing in the doorway at home waiting for the celebrity gimp. Aunt Naomi was wearing a kinda frumpy housedress with some kind of small print on it. Joel wore the uniform he and the Kid had worn ever since they'd been living together: DeeCee overalls and a shirt Aunt Naomi had made from a flour sack.

A big smile from Joel which went all the way through to the Kid's belly. A big hug from Aunt Naomi which felt just as good, maybe even better. And the bed where he held court for the next two days as kith and kin came to get their first look at the Kid who had polio and lived to talk about it. And to express some genuine concern. Or maybe to steal some of the Kid's comic books which he'd brought home. And he'd brought home a hundred or more stacked up a yard high.

The Kid could hear the grownups asking all kinds of questions to satisfy their morbid curiosity about the effects of the viri. "How bad off is he now? Will he ever be normal again? Will he be able to walk? Will he need braces or crutches or a wheelchair? Has he gotten any better since you took him to Memphis? What are y'all gonna do about all this? It's too much a burden to ask y'all to cope with, ain't it? He's not your child, you shouldn't have to be stuck with this. I think it's just awful that nobody else has stepped in and took over. It's not like it was Joel."

The Kid's ears had not been adversely affected by the viri. He heard what they said. And he wasn't sure whether they gave a good goddamn whether he heard or not. Uncle Sam and Aunt Naomi stuck in there, though, albeit often very reluctantly, probably because they thought people would think it would be in bad taste if they just dropped the Kid off alongside the road—in a park, perhaps—like dad had done with Snowball.

But it was obvious they weren't thrilled about being gimp-sitters for the son of the drunken adulterer. Besides, money was tight and it was a fact that trips to Memphis for checkups and treatment and the cost of special equipment and support shoes and the like was higher than they could afford for *their own* and the fact that the Kid wasn't, really, added to their quandary.

Christmas Day was at grandmother's house in Paris. The ten mile trip was sunny and pleasant. The Kid felt like he could jump out of the car just like he had on that last Friday before Thanksgiving when he'd been picking corn. After more than four weeks in the hospital, simply being on the outside of a building was a joy!

Watching the birds sitting on light wires and fences all along the Mansfield Road. Watching soft white puffs of clouds play touch football. The sound of Aunt Naomi's voice as she talked quietly to Uncle Sam. The sight of Joel jostling alongside him in the backseat. Perhaps there was Nirvana after the log house on Whitlock Road. Perhaps.

Uncle Sam carried him up the steps and across the long front porch at grandmother's house into the living room and onto her couch which had been made into a sickbed especially for the occasion. The Kid was gonna get hisself some attention today and he was up to it.

Suddenly the Kid, who had mostly attracted attention all his life by being a pain in the ass, was the center of everybody's oohing and aahing. Sympathy was everywhere. People who normally wouldn't pay the slightest attention to him walked up to him first thing when they came into the house to get their very first look at a polio person. Yeah, he might look like the Kid, but you could tell he wasn't.

The viri had changed everything. This poor little feller couldn't hardly move, much less walk. He'd been a month in that big ole hospital in Memphis and he was going to go back again the day after Christmas. Poor little guy. Polio done knocked the meanness out of him. Left him a little spoiled maybe but very sweet.

Grandmother's house was heated by a grate, a small fireplace that burned coal instead of wood and took up less room than a big wood-burning fireplace and hearth. The center of the rough wooden floor was covered with a linoleum rug whose design was worn almost all the way through to the tarpaper or whatever it was that linoleum really was. Around the edges of the rug was furniture polished to a high shine.

Granddaddy's comfortable platform rocker was in the corner. A convertible couch sat between the outside door and the door to the spare bedroom. On walls hung wartime pictures of Uncle Sam and Uncle Pete in their uniforms. Those pictures in their ornate oval wooden frames were grandmother's pride and joy.

Uncle Sam was the "best boy there ever wuz until he went to that ole war. The best there ever could be." Where Uncle Sam had been absolutely perfect Uncle Pete had only been almost absolutely perfect, suffering perhaps a loss of a tenth of a point or so for his lack of great height. He was short. But he was wonderful. "Almost from the day Pete could walk he worked. Like a dog. When he was five or six years old he'd walk behind Elmore's mule, pushing a plow. He couldn't hardly reach the crossbar and had to tie the reins behind his neck because he couldn't steer the plow and the mules at the same time. And I mean did a good job!"

But for one day in the house that glowed from the shine of Uncle Sam and Uncle Pete, the Kid was the star. All obeisance to the Kid. And gifts. Toys of every description from everybody. Peggy gave him a really neat wallet. Dollar bills had to be folded in half before they would fit. Small enough for a seven year old in a hospital. Somebody gave him a real watch which he would remember three years later when somebody gave him a toy watch for his tenth birthday.

Actually, the watch lasted several days before he was compelled to investigate its origins and workings and found it inestimably more difficult to put it back together again than it had been to take it apart.

And when the giving had turned to trash he wasn't ready to quit. "Is that all I got? I want more. I didn't get enough yet." It felt like he hurt Peggy's feelings when he said that, although he hadn't intended to. He didn't even know why he'd said it. Except that getting stuff had felt so good.

Going to the toilet wasn't so wonderful. Legs that didn't work couldn't take him to the outside john grand-daddy had built down by the garden. Arms that didn't work couldn't unbutton overall pants. Uncle Sam had to do it all for him including the zipping and unzipping and diggling and jiggling.

The house was full that Christmas Day: mom's siblings their spouses and children; Aunt Louise, dad's sister, with Uncle Nolan and their children; the home bunch, Peggy, Jacky and Ronald. And maybe more.

While the adults sat around the dining table in the kitchen Peggy brought the Kid's dinner into the living room: baked chicken, cornbread dressing and gravy, mashed potatoes, fried corn, string beans, cornbread, bis-cuits, apple pie, custard pie.

Grandmother couldn't cook worth a shit, but the Kid didn't know that then. The Kid didn't know that for years. Grandmother would spoil him forever with her leathery-tough biscuits. Who wanted those fluffy cakes of air when there were those flat chewy wonderful biscuits that could also be used as weapons in an emergency?

But it wouldn't be just grandmother's cooking that would catch and hold onto the Kid's attention for years afterward: Aunt Margaret's and Aunt Lillian's po-tato salad and Uncle Sam's chili that was so hot that it made his hair stand on end. From then on unless chili

94

made his hair stand on end the Kid would dismiss it as unchili. A marvelous Christmas feast in nineteen-fifty.

Too soon, though, it was over. And back to Uncle Sam's and into bed. Til the morrow when the body had to be returned to Isolation Hospital.

This time they didn't stop Uncle Sam at the door. He walked all the way to the Kid's floor and stood by, watching, while others pushed the Kid on a stretcher to his room and lifted the Kid to his bed. And watched the Kid's eyes widen to the size of saucers when he saw a stack of presents there. More Christmas. Lots more Christmas.

Recognizing an ideal exit time when he saw it, Uncle Sam split before the Kid cared whether he was gone.

The big box was a set of holsters and cap pistols. Two gun draw. Just like Roy Rogers. Even better than the Kid had had when he lived in the log house. Books. Games. Clothes.

The Shriners and the Kiwanians and the Elks and just about every other civic organization in town looking for feel-good giving had dropped off gifts. More gifts than all the gifts the Kid had received at grandmother's house yesterday.

His girlfriend in the respirator smiled at the joy on her young friend's face. Yes, she had gotten her share of gifts. And more. Seeing her made him glow. He was sorry when she disappeared two days later. A nurse said she had gone home and taken her respirator with her.

The Kid never believed she went home unless it was a Jesus thing they were talking about and, if so, why would she need a respirator up there?

He saw an extra respirator in the hallway shortly afterwards. The Kid knew his friend had died. He knew she had gone away and he equated disappearance with death. Half a century later the Kid in all his maturity had advanced his notion much further.

Death is disappearance.

Hopalong Cassidy

The new year also brought a pleasant change to the Kid's world, although it didn't seem so at the time. He was transferred to Crippled Children's Hospital in Memphis, the rehab hospital for children of the viri and of the cerebral palsy and sometimes of the burns. A stranger, an African-American man, pushed a stretcher into his room one morning in January of nineteen-fifty-one. "Hey, I'm Leon. I come to take you to a new home."

The Kid froze with fear. *What did he mean a new home? The only home he had besides Uncle Sam's was here at Isolation Hospital.*

"I'm not supposed to go anywhere."

"Oh yes you are. Don't be afraid. You're gonna really like Crippled Children's Hospital. And I'm gonna drive you over there in a station wagon. You ever been in a station wagon? That'll be a lot of fun."

The nurse who'd followed Leon into the room smiled as she nodded. "He's right Kid. There'll be lots more to do over at Crippled Children's. They've got TV and movies and you can go to school. You're going to love it there. I promise this is nothing to be scared of. You trust me, don't you?"

Nod.

"Okay."

Tears falling gently down his cheeks. *Something awful's going to happen. It's going to hurt. I know it is. They're going to hurt me.*

97

She helped Leon pull the Kid onto the stretcher, hugged him and patted him on the head as he disappeared through the door into the corridor.

It was not a short trip down to the station wagon. Although Leon had pointed it out to the Kid from the window where it sat in the parking lot it was a helluva lot further away than it looked. Leon transferred the Kid from the hospital stretcher to one inside the back of the station wagon, slammed the back door shut, jumped into the driver's side, started the engine and lit a cigarette.

"Here we go. It's a beautiful day for a drive, isn't it?" And they drove through the biggest city the Kid had ever seen. Everywhere there were people and huge buildings and big streets and bustling sidewalks and trees and automobiles and neon signs. *Wow! Wow! Wow!* Exclamations were all that could even begin to describe the wonder the Kid felt as he and Leon plied the streets of Memphis town. *Wow! Everybody here is rich! Wow!* Kids running and jumping everywhere first excited and then saddened the Kid as he realized that that wasn't something he could do anymore, not anymore like in the old days with Jacky.

"Over there is the zoo." Leon pointed down a long tree-lined walkway. "Ever been to a zoo?"

"Uh uh."

"But you'd like to go, I bet, wouldn't you?"

"Uh huh."

"Yeah. All them lions 'n tigers 'n elephants 'n kangaroos. They got bears in there with mouths big enuf to eatchoo wif one big bite. Sho' nuf!"

Eventually Leon turned the Ford right onto a side street and then left into a driveway that ran along the back of a large two-storied brick building. "We're home," he announced with a big smile as he gestured grandly with his left hand through the open window.

The Kid was scared. Again. At the moment he wasn't sure that he wouldn't be safer with that big-mouthed bear than inside this strange building with all those people who were surely going to cause him more pain. He was sure that every one of them had a big needle, just waiting for him to come by so they could jab him wherever it hurt the worst. Whatever awaited him he knew it wasn't pleasant.

"What you shaking for, boy?" Leon grinned in what he probably thought was a friendly gesture but which to the Kid covered up the terror that awaited him inside the doors of that building. "They gonna treat choo good in here. Ain't nobody gonna hurt choo one little bit. You'll really like it here. Really."

Leon disappeared through the doors to reappear almost immediately rolling a stretcher to the back door of the station wagon. "Here ya go," he said, as he opened the door and pulled the Kid gently from the vehicle onto the sheet covering the cold metal top of the stretcher. Into the mouth of the evil dragon through the double doors, down the green corridor to the big elevator with its scissoring latticework door.

The elevator, in truth, was a magical manipulator of time, making a fifteen second ride from the basement to the first floor seem like hours to the Kid, hours to compound the dread of what surely would come when they discovered he was here.

Off the elevator, Leon pushed the Kid past a large room on the right filled with kids laughing and talking and eating. "That's the dining room," pointed Leon. "That's where all the kids go when they're able to get out of bed for their meals."

Left into another green-colored corridor. To its end. Through a big doorway into a huge room filled with big baby beds just like the one the Kid had been in for the last couple of months over at Isolation Hospital. About half of the beds were empty.

Leon pulled the stretcher to a stop. "Where's this boy's bed?" he called out.

"That middle one over there on the left. Two up from where you are."

Satan, disguised as a woman dressed in white, walked over. *This is it. She's the one that's gonna get me. Help me. Send somebody to help me before she can hurt me. Oh no! Ooooooh!*

"Is this our new patient? Are you the Kid? My name is Miss Bean and I'll be taking care of you."

You're goin' t' hurt me. I know it.

She took the stretcher from Leon and pushed it between two beds snugging it up against one with the barred side lowered. "Help me here, Leon. I'll get on the other side and pull. You come here and give him a shove." The bed smelled like a hospital bed — the scent of painted iron. It also smelled like wash day. Like the sheets had just come off the clothesline before they'd been tucked so carefully onto the bed. The bottom sheet stretched tautly over the mattress pad; the top sheet folded back two-thirds of the way toward the foot of the bed and tucked tightly under the mattress so it would

100

look decent until it was needed. Then it pulled up like unfolding an accordion, although accordions that flat and freshly starched look fairly unused.

He was on the bed. It smelled good.

Miss Bean pulled up the bars on both sides of the bed to half-mast. The Kid felt his fear disappear. Not only would the bars keep him from going anywhere, as long as they were up they would protect him from the needles and hoses and sundry harassments plied by the practicing medicine men and women.

"You got here just in time for lunch. Everybody's just about finished but when we heard you were coming we saved enough back for you. Are you hungry?" He nodded tentatively. "Okay, if you'll turn over you can eat now." Miss Bean set a tray on the mattress after the Kid had turned over and raised himself up onto his elbows. "Here's some nice spinach and potatoes and milk." *Looks better than food at Isolation. Maybe this place won't be so bad after all.* He dug in. *Yech!* The spinach didn't taste a thing like turnip greens or mustard greens. It tasted like it was rotten. And that cheese on top. *This is awful.* The tomatoes were the first hothouse tomatoes the Kid had ever tasted. They were pretty bad, too, but after the bottom of the toilet taste of the spinach not too bad to eat. So he ate them. And the potatoes and white bread and jello. And milk.

"You didn't eat your spinach. We all clean our plates here, Kid. We can't throw away good food. But since this is your first day I suppose we can let you slip by with this. Just don't let it happen again. Now be a good boy and take your nap. Twelve o'clock to two o'clock is nap time here. Everybody has to take a nap. That's the rules. Everybody, so don't feel like you're being treated any different than anybody else. Here, let me pull your sheet up over you. Naptime means no talking, no playing games or reading. Naptime means taking a nap. You can meet the rest of the boys later. You'll have plenty of time to get acquainted and get in trouble while we're fixing you up so you can get out of here. Now go to sleep."

"Who are you?" The Kid turned his head to the left toward the source of the whispered query. "Kid," he answered, keeping his voice as quiet as he could to avoid the wrath he was sure Miss Bean would rain down on him if she caught him breaking her rules. "I'm Ronnie Lane. Where you from?" "Mansfield." "I'm from Camden. We'd better not talk anymore. Miss Bean don't like talking during nap time. Talk to you later."

Crippled Children's Hospital would become the Kid's all-time favorite childhood home.

Aside from the terrible cheese and spinach and other stuff he hated so bad, the food was good. Cereal for breakfast every morning except Sunday when they had bacon and eggs and toast. Spaghetti and meatballs every Saturday for lunch. Hamburgers once a week. Buttery stewed potatoes once a week for supper with all the white bread you wanted to eat. It was heaven.

Movies twice a week. Real movies on Wednesday night and Saturday afternoon. Just like the ones in the movie theaters. A lot of adventure stories which satisfied the Kid just fine. Saturday movies were old westerns and serials like they used to show at the Princess. The Kid was thrilled to see Captain Marvel's new adventures and the whole Marvel family. But the best were the cowboy movies.

Hopalong Cassidy all dressed up in black, riding Topper. Bill Boy dressed up in khaki. Bill Boy and Hopalong Cassidy were played by the same actor whose screen name was William Boyd. The Kid wondered about that sometimes, but didn't let befuddlement get between him and a good time. Lash LaRue. Tim Holt. Rex Allen. Tex Ritter. There were dozens of cowboy stars and hundreds of crooks for them to shoot and fight and jail.

The movies were shown in the auditorium which had a kitchen attached. And inside the kitchen was a popcorn popper. Just like the one they had at the Princess Theater in Paris. Good popcorn, that. Good popcorn.

Kids who could walk, walked to the auditorium and sat in chairs in front of the kids who were in wheelchairs in front of the stretcher regiment of beds — the patients who weren't allowed out of bed — bringing up the royal rear.

There were three wards in the hospital: the boys, the girls, and the babies. Events like the movies provided an opportunity for some intermingling of the opposite sexes, although most of them didn't know what the hell that meant, anyhow. They just knew it felt good and that was okay.

The Kid knew it meant something else and he'd been trying to figure that out for years, ever since he'd gotten those fuzzy feelings for Annie Catherine, but he wasn't any further ahead in the figuring than the completely unaware.

He had more friends than he had time to keep up with. Ronnie Lane was his best buddy. They always tried to have their beds parked next to each other whenever they went into the auditorium for special events. After awhile the Kid felt more secure in the rehab hospital in the care of professionals than he had felt since before his mom had been killed by Sam Garrett in the movie he'd both hated and replayed the most.

Every ward had its own television set, mounted over the door opening into the corridor. There were strict rules about watching television. Only the nurse could turn it on or change the channels, although some of the more agile patients, and those who were tall enough, learned quickly how to push a chair over and make adjustments.

TV viewing started with Howdy Doody time and continued pretty much uninterrupted until eight o'clock lights out. The Kid had never watched television before. In his life. This was the ultimate adventure for him. A cornucopia of experiences. Buffalo Bob and Clara Bell and Snuffy Smith and good ole Howdy. And the kids in the peanut gallery.

During the day every ward had its own nurse. Nurse was a misnomer. They were nurses to the kids but what they were in real life were nurse's "aides". Whatever they were called, they were the surrogate parents of the people under their care. And treated that way by their charges.

The aides were the ruler of the roost. They stopped short of paddling their patients — that was left to the hospital director who scared the bejeezus out of everyone so badly that actual paddling almost never occurred — but he didn't hesitate to scare the shit out of them to keep them in line. And did a remarkable job considering how many kids they each had to deal with and considering that each kid had an unbelievable amount of pent up energy resulting from close quarters confinement, often for months, sometimes for years, between the onset of his/her disease and transfer to rehab.

The older kids were more likely to fall in serious infatuation with the aides they liked best. And they did. Often.

Within days of his arrival the Kid was enrolled in the second grade. "You've been on vacation too long, Kid." The teacher was Miss Graves who was an old time polio veteran herself. She looked like she was a hundred to the Kid which means she was probably somewhere on the downside of fifty, seeing as how most post-polios didn't live into their sixties back then. She was a tiny bent-over lady who walked around with the help of one crutch under her right arm. Giving her freedom to perform miracles with the left.

Gentle Miss Graves with bobbed grey-mixed-with-white hair who, not unlike some benevolent frankensteinian monster, could be detected from many feet away far down the corridor by the staccato arrhythmic repetition of shoe-crutch-shoe-crutch-shoe-crutch, almost like a macabre skipping misstep dance.

Miss Graves would be the catalyst for kicking the Kid into real studentdom, seeking real information and answers. 'Course polio had its effect in that area, too; if you can't walk or run or play with the normal kids in a normal setting, you play in your mind and the visions begin with reading.

And the Kid started doing a whole lot of reading after the evil viri got him. Before he had devoted himself almost exclusively to running and jumping and hunting and wandering and climbing and folding himself up inside car tires for cartwheeling.

Miss Graves tutored the Kid through the second grade, the last half of the sixth grade and all of the seventh. She raised her voice in exasperation exactly once during all those tens of hundreds of hours. Miss Graves was mild-mannered. And caring. And a damn good teacher. Actually, the Kid had been pretty lucky in roulette pick of the teacher crop since the beginning. Miss Pillow at Puryear's first grade was a tall Miss Graves except she couldn't spend as much time with the Kid or any other single student because she had a classful on her hands.

Miss Graves sang her soothing song to the young punk who could only be conquered by the evil viri before he'd listen to any teacher.

At first the Kid didn't move so well and couldn't get out of bed, so she'd bring his workbooks and assignments to the ward in the morning and pick them up in the afternoon, grade them and have them back the next morning. The Kid didn't have anything better to do with his time so he started paying attention and getting decent grades.

Miss Graves didn't make anybody work very hard. And she didn't give anybody bad grades unless they were totally hopeless and the Kid never saw or heard about a one of them. School work became fun. Mostly workbooks with lessons and questions. Infrequent tests and then, as never before, the testee was adequately prepared. She gave a shit. There are far worse legacies.

When the kids were allowed to be moved, they congregated in the auditorium for morning and afternoon classes where there were fewer distractions. Miss Graves would go from bed to chair to desk picking up assignments, handling out explanations, encouraging and fussing about how everybody could always do better than they thought.

"You're not only as good as you think you are," she would say, "you're a whole lot better than that. There is no one here who can't be an A-plus student. But you've got to learn to do it on your own. I'm not always going to be here to hold your hand and wipe your eyes and give you easy tests and good grades. You're going to have to do it yourselves."

Then you'd see her furrowed brow metamorphose into one of those infectious grins. She wasn't, however, without a temper. On more than one occasion the Kid shuddered with apprehension when he heard her crutch-shoes skipping across the floor, getting closer and closer, after he'd failed to do his work, or, just as bad, after he'd given his work short shrift.

The dark eyebrows started their wrinkling as soon as she spotted her prey and hunched closer and closer until she was within earshot which was when she loosed the arrows she'd dipped in venom and irritation. 'Twas a rare arrow that missed its mark. 'Twas a rare occasion that study habits and homework didn't improve after one of her patented shooting matches.

Then Mrs. Norcross, the book lady, started stopping by his bed every week and he started reading. Mrs. Norcross collected books from all over and gave them to Crippled Children patients. Not borrow. Not lend. Not pay back. Gave. Yours forever or until you turn a funny color. Ownership does something for the reader's soul. And it did for the Kid. First the comic books. Not just any comics, the book lady only brought "classic" comic books: Ivanhoe, Tale of Two Cities, The Man in the Iron Mask, The Hunchback of Notre Dame.

Suddenly a new world started opening for the Kid. Other benefactors brought other kinds of comic books: Archie and Donald Duck and the like, and he took them, but his pride was the collection of classic comics. Half a century later he can revisit the eagerness he felt when the book lady came through the door of the ward, wondering what she would have today to add to his collection.

The comic books led to reading books that didn't contain any pictures: Hardy Brothers and Nancy Drew and the Bobsy Twins, all teenage detectives. The Kid's life as a reader was like a rollercoaster that starts off very, very slowly as it is pulled up the steep slope. Slowly. Oh so slowly. Hesitates for a microsecond at the top. Then plunges into the adventure of the ride, gathering speed, and giggles.

The Kid's still hanging onto the side of that old claptrap coaster with its infrastructure's crumbling wood. The cars are bare metal, skinned of their showy paint jobs by the sunshine and eager hands caressing their sides as they've made a million rides on the uphill side. But they ain't done yet. Not while there's still juice and baling wire to keep it from collapsing in on itself. Creak. Creak.

The triumphant triumvirate. Mrs. Norcross and Miss Graves and the evil viri. The Kid is a reader, tried and true, proud and pure, til he dies.

School was just about the funnest thing for the Kid at Crippled Children. And the food. And the movies. And the books. And the kids. And Miss Bean the mommy figure.

Hot Packs and Jesus

Not everything, however, was a barrel of laughs. Torture was not far away from any point in the day, except usually the Kid could rest easy after lights out. First thing they hit him with at Crippled Children was hot baths. HOT baths. The afternoon aide would strip his clothes off, pick him up and take him into the bathroom where a tub filled with three or four inches of steaming hot water awaited. And she'd stick his body in there, heedless of the screams that emanated. She'd gently lower his head onto a block of wood that served as a pillow to keep him from drowning as well as boiling.

Someone later said one-hundred-eight degrees. He knew it was scalding him. Day after day. Right after supper. The Kid hated for supper to be over. One night she forgot to come back to turn the water off. It was up to his chin and hotter than it usually was by the time she remembered and came running.

A cauldron of special witches brew designed to replicate the pain a missionary would go through while he's being cooked for dinner in a neighboring cannibal's village.

Heat was thought to be an effective medium for restoring muscle control in post-polio people.

Just as the Kid was learning to endure the hot water they hit him with "hot packs". A hot pack is a strip of woolen blanket which has been heated in boiling water in a special cooker. When it reaches the desired temperature, the cooker goes through a kind of tumbling cycle where most of the water is centrifuged from the wool without significantly reducing the temperature.

As soon as the tumbling stops, the aide opens the lid, carefully staying a bit back to avoid the cloud of steam spewing from it, dips a pair of long-handled tongs inside and brings out a nice boiling-hot piece of wool which she rushes over to the victim. She then wraps the wool around the afflicted part of the victim's anatomy and immediately covers it with insulating material to keep it hot and plastic to keep the bed relatively dry while the victim is shrieking in pain caused by the extreme heat.

At first the Kid screamed and cried aloud every time someone approached him with a hot pack; he required them from his ankles to his neck, including his arms, so he was almost totally covered with them.

Later, he cried and shrieked silently, not wanting to appear to be cowardly when it seemed like everyone else in the ward was taking their steaming wool with aplomb. Two to five times a day. Until the wool cooled to a durable temperature. Then they'd do it all over again.

There was a method to applying the hot packs at just the right temperature, which was tolerable when they were cooler, but which actually burned, blistering the skin, when they were hotter. Eventually those blisters were just one more thing to endure, often coming at the hands of the same aide who was either a sadist, incompetent, or stupidly thought the hotter the better, regardless of medicinal efficacy.

Some of them would even continue applying the hot packs over the blisters without bringing them to the attention of the LPN or the RN until they were ordered to cease and desist by a doctor who examined the patients weekly or one of the nurses who spot checked for blisters.

The blisters were actually counterproductive because they disrupted the prescribed treatment program. Once they were spotted, that part of the patient's body was allowed to heal before the torture continued.

It's needless to say that polio patients did not enjoy the hot pack-filled days, and were, in fact, scared mostly half to death.

Imagine being paralyzed, which is traumatic in itself. Then imagine being jerked away from your family. Imagine being suddenly stuck with a bunch of strangers, many of whom regularly inflict severe pain on you. Imagine further the terror anticipation of that pain builds inside your child's mind. Now imagine yourself as that terrorized, pain wracked, helpless child who has absolutely no defense against whatever anyone who can move and get to him wants to do with him.

Can you imagine that?

The Kid never had to use his imagination. *They're coming to get me. He He Ha Ha! They're coming to get me. Ha Ha!* And they did. "This won't hurt much, Kid. I promise!" Yeah and what's the song about it don't rain in Indianapolis in the summer time? And little green apples? Yeah!

There was always prayer to pull him out, now wasn't there? Didn't he have to say the blessing before every meal?

"God is great,
God is good.
Let us thank Him
for our food.
Amen."

There! There! Isn't that better?

111

"It's lights out, boys. Don't forget your prayers. I'll say them with you."

"Now I lay me down to sleep
I pray the Lord my soul to keep
If I should die before I wake
I pray the Lord my soul to take
Amen."

Aaah, the night. Once again to be able to cuddle in the arms of the Lord who had avowed to protect the Kid and all the rest of the kids in the ward against evil and evildoers while the lights were out.

Apparently God slept during the day when the shit hit the hot pack machines. Couldn't expect the poor guy to be everywhere. Right? The little man who brought Sunday School to the hospital was certain, though, that Jesus loved everybody and was going to take good care of them, if not in this world, then in the next.

"It's not for us to second-guess why things happen to us the way they do. All we know is that they're in God's greater plan. We only know we'll understand it better by and by when the roll is called up yonder in the city where the streets are all paved with gold and where there's no more pain or sadness."

"Doesn't that sound good, boys and girls? Won't it be wonderful when Jesus brings us home to that city in heaven where we won't ever again have to worry about anything?"

"Won't it be wonderful?"

"All we have to do is believe in the Lord Jesus Christ and thou shalt be saved."

"Let us sing:

> Jesus loves the little children
> all the little children of the world
> red and yellow, black and white
> they are precious in His sight
> Jesus loves the little children of the world."

"I know a lot of you are suffering in this world below. I want you to know that I pray for you every day. Don't forget your prayers. Jesus hears every one of them. He answers every one of your prayers. Whether you like the answer or not, He does answer every one of them. And He loves you."

The Kid thought it was kinda strange that if Jesus loved everybody so much and had His eye on the sparrow and cared so much about helping people out, how He sat back and didn't do jackshit when the nurses or their aides slapped those burning hot packs on his body. Or when they eased his body down into the boiling water every night. Or when Doctor Ingram came in and showed all his student doctors just how bad polio could hurt.

The Kid thought Jesus and God must be pretty strange to give a shit and never act like it.

Unless you counted letting them live. Was that the blessing? Yeh! Had to be. Okay, now it's all clear. Don't matter if they pitch you in a vat of boiling water long as you survive it.

Not long after the hot packs made their debut, the physical therapist walked over to the Kid's bed. "It's time to start our exercises," she said as she pressed her right hand against his knees and pulled his head down with her left until his nose was touching his extended knee.

113

The Kid started screaming about the time she got his torso into a sitting position. By the time she'd pushed his head all the way down between his knees the pain was beyond screaming. He was speechless. Only every fiber of every muscle in his whole body was still screaming. Silently.

Just when he thought it couldn't get any worse it did.

"I know it hurts, but you'll get used to it before you know it."

Three more times. *Why won't they leave me alone? I can't stand this pain. And I can't run away. Ooooooooooooooh. Ooooooooooooooh!* Tears were to no avail. She'd seen too many of them. Besides, nothing would keep her from the course.

It was the first time since the previous November the Kid had sat. He wasn't real eager to do it again. Ever. At that cost.

"I'll be coming in every day, Kid, to limber you up with these exercises. So you might as well dry up those tears and get used to it. It is for your own good. Straighten up and act like the man you can be."

She was about as big as a minute. Skinny as a rail. Small arms covered with wrinkled skin. Gray hair. With a grip that Jesus couldn't break even if He hadn't been sleeping at that time of the day.

That wasn't the end of it. Bowel movements. A bowel movement every day, or else. Else was you'd get a shot glass filled with mineral oil. Castor oil is its nearest relative. So thick it's almost not liquid. Makes you wanna puke. But you can't. If you puke, you get another one. And another and another until you don't puke. So the

114

boys almost never puked. The boys tried never not to have a bowel movement every day. There was no way they could fake it.

Bed patients used bedpans which told the story which the aide could then report on the daily BM chart. If the patient was a walker he'd wait until the aide checked the toilet before he flushed so she could make a report. One deranged kid got so hungry while he waited for someone to come by and check that he had some of his bowel movement for a late snack! (*My dear FL: you said in your preface that some of your stories may be figments of your imagination. I think this one fits the category. -- CB*)

Walking Any Walk

Patients of Crippled Children's Hospital were, for the most part, people with polio or cerebral palsy (CP). Their length of stay averaged several months. They were sent there to learn to function in the outside world, by which they would forevermore be deemed outsiders, the best they could. Those persons with CP were generally in the baby ward since their handicaps occurred at birth, which allowed their habilitation (rehabilitation implies previous non-gimpness which CP people did not have) to start early, as soon as they were old enough to learn to walk and feed themselves.

They were the group that had the heavy full-leg braces from shoes to waist walkers. They spent much of their days in physical therapy trying to learn basic coping skills. They had a long way to go from admission to discharge. When those leg braces came off they crumbled like wet toilet paper. The only thing keeping their legs erect were those braces. Most of them were so thin and seemed to be so weak the Kid wondered how they found the strength to move the braces at all. This was before the advent of strong aluminum.

Many of the braces were steel and leather. Steel going up the lower leg to the knee where it was jointed to another piece of steel going up to the hip where it was jointed with a leather and steel girdle which strapped around the waist. The knee joints had slip locks to freeze them in an extended position. The locks were short pieces of steel that could be pushed over the ends of both upper and lower leg staves, making the knee joint immobile. The knees were covered with leather that attached to the brace. And there were leather straps that encircled the upper and lower legs.

It was tough for those persons with CP. Often upon admission they were not able to do much more than sit and then only in a crazy kind of fluid way with no ability to stabilize in any position. Softly flailing the air with hands and arms and legs and feet. They could not feed themselves or do much of anything for themselves. The saddest part of it is that they could not, in the vast majority, communicate with most people. Perhaps to a limited degree with their parents and other family members, but in the hospital they were held incommunicado by a handicap that is often caused by the medical community screwing up at birth. The ultimate imprisonment.

Many of them did improve significantly over many months. Many of them did learn to walk and sit relatively straight — sometimes with a corset — and feed themselves. And some of them beat seemingly insurmountable odds to find success — whatever that meant to them — in life. Most, however, could not pass through their formidable barriers to happy ever after.

Aside from the terror, the Kid oddly found comfort in the homey atmosphere of Crippled Children's Hospital. In addition to the aides there were several maids working at bathing the children and assisting the aides. The maids were, without exception, African-American.

The Kid would wake up in the morning when the maid turned on the lights at six o'clock to get the day started with tooth brushing. Mrs. Deming, the overnight aide, put toothpaste on brushes and carried the toothbrushes, metal spit basins and metal cups for rinsing around to the beds in the hospital before the end of her shift. The cups all had a patient's name printed with ballpoint pen on a piece of what had once been white tape. While the boys were brushing their teeth the metal urinals would be collected, emptied, cleaned, and returned. Then collection of the brushes, basins and cups.

Time for breakfast. There was one maid per ward. Each would take a big cart on wheels and push it down to the dumbwaiter on the far side of the dining room and stack trays for the kids who had to eat in the ward. Once the bed patients were given their trays the maid took the walkers and wheelchair mobile to the dining room for their corn flakes and toast. Or, if it was a good day, Rice Krispies. Big post-polio kids who could use their arms helped feed the CP kids who couldn't.

Because milk and cereal usually wound up on just about everybody, bathing was reserved until afterwards. Also because that was the time the aides came on duty, eight o'clock, which meant more help, especially for those who couldn't bathe themselves.

Actually there were three groups of baths in the boys ward: tub baths for those who were mobile and who didn't have body parts that had to be protected from water, as with severe burns; self-administered sponge baths for patients who were old enough and mobile enough but who couldn't get out of bed and into a bathtub; and sponge baths for patients administered by maids and aides because the patients were either too young to do it themselves or simply could not sufficiently move the body parts they would have needed to move to get the job done.

The Kid especially enjoyed being sponge bathed by the pretty aides and maids. One thing for sure, the evil viri didn't close down his fledgling libido one little bit.

The Kid would never grow up. He got older, but he never got over loving to look at pretty aides and maids. All in a row. Or not.

After breakfast, the maids cleaned the floor; the aides cleaned and made the beds just like they'd been taught in boot camp.

Hot pack time. Steam the muscles loose til ten. Make way for the physical therapist who shoved his nose between his knees up to twenty times without quitting. And more hot packs to get him well done by lunchtime.

Naptime. Each bed had a footboard stuck upright between the frame and the mattress. Prisoners of the evil viri were required, as part and parcel of their daily torture, to press their feet flat—with legs outstretched—against the board. Hard. This was supposed to be the rule whenever they were in bed, but the inspectors paid special attention at nap and night time.

Otherwise, oh, what a wonderful two hours when the Kid tried to read. Tried, but got caught just about every day by Miss Bean who grabbed his book from him. "No reading. Not for you or anyone else, Kid. You know I can't play favorites." The Kid knew that he was one of her very favorite patients anyway. He liked how it felt. Like snuggling in a warm blanket.

Hot packs after the nap. More physical therapist bumping his knees with his nose.

In fairly short order the Kid was introduced to occupational therapy which would turn out to be his happiest time of the day—if you don't count the movies and movie stars. Occupational therapy was another kind of physical therapy, except trickier. Mrs. Robinson was the therapist. Her job was to help the patients regain the use of their fine motor skills. She had lots and lots of fascinating projects to help them along the way, none of which looked like exercise. None of which was scary at all.

Painting pictures by number was fun. Sewing leather wallets together with laces, using increasingly difficult knots, was fascinating. Making lanyards, potholders, belts. Most of the patients could hardly wait for Mrs. Robinson to bring her goody-filled cart around in the afternoon for another session of making something for somebody at home.

Swimming was stuck in the afternoon, usually between occupational therapy and dinner. So the swimmers wouldn't get a tummy ache, I guess. The Kid, who had always loved the water, took to this like an old duck. Yeah, seven would be old for a duck. He had never even seen a swimming pool before, indoor or outdoor, and here was this huge concrete hole inside the hospital filled with warm, inviting water.

And a bonus; at Crippled Children's Hospital they taught him how to swim. Really swim. On his back. Or his belly.

At first the physical therapist in charge would take the Kid down to the pool on a stretcher, lift him gently and walk with him in her arms into the water. Before he thought it was great, however, he was scared half out of his wits. He had always splashed about with his arms and legs and managed to keep moving toward fun and games with Jacky.

Now that he could hardly move his arms the water was no longer a friend to visit. It had become a dreadful enemy lying in wait to pump his lungs full of water and push him down, down, down! Until he died a ghastly death. He'd seen it happen often enough in his comic books that he knew what was in store for him if the therapist let go for more than a second or two. And so, when she did let go, he let go with a scream that started in the core of his soul, gaining momentum as it wended its way to the outside world.

"Help! I can't. I'll drown!"

It was several weeks before he could control his hysteria sufficiently to follow the simplest instructions. Gradually, however, the water once again became his friend. He could float on his back for as long as he wanted to. No way he could drown as long as he could float, was there? And he could swim on his back, even if his right leg hung uselessly toward the bottom. He could swim on his belly, even if his left leg couldn't kick backwards. But he could swim! He could hardly wait to show his cousins in the lake back home after he got out. Swimming came to be one of the most enjoyable forms of exercise the Kid would ever know.

Supper was served at the hospital at four-thirty, about the same time the wardens allowed the television set to be turned on. It didn't matter to the Kid what program was on. He loved to look at the little box with the flickering picture. And he loved to eat. He especially loved doing both at the same time.

After supper was free time when the patients were able to do whatever they wanted to do as long as they "followed the rules". Some played cards. Others read books Mrs. Norcross had brought them. Wheelchair patients chased each other up and down the ward and, when the aide wasn't looking, into the hallway where they weren't allowed.

Sometimes, when the aide was on a mission away from the ward, the wheelchair gang would venture afield, going as far as the babies' ward at the opposite end of the hallway. Where they were inevitably caught and herded back in a shower of sundry reprimands streaming volubly from the pretty mouth sitting atop the open collar of that swishy white nylon dress.

The aide was the most important part of the nighttime games. Everything depended on her cooperation. Two bed patients could only get together to play if she would lower one side of each bed and push them together. Wheelchair patients needed her approval for them to stay up in their wheelchairs in order for them to move around in the circle of fun and games which was the highlight of their days.

Seven o'clock was lights out for the babies' ward. The boys and girls could keep theirs on until eight.

Then. Lights out. No more games. No talking. No whispering. No making noise of any kind. Quiet. Everyone settled down under the blue glow of "germ lights", special bulbs mounted in fixtures where the ceiling met the wall. Several in each ward. Light which looked a lot like ultraviolet. Supposed to protect against bad germs? The Kid knew they called them "germ lights" and that they barely gave off enough light for him to read by. Which might explain why he had to have glasses early on. If eye strain and poor vision are connected.

He'd have a book or two tucked away in his bed bag for sneaking out after lights out. A bed bag was a cloth bag which was tied to the bars at the head of the bed. It held the patient's "important" stuff. And was important for patients who could not reach their bedside tables because of the work of the evil viri. He read himself to sleep or until his eyes hurt too much to continue.

What a wonderful escape from the often brutal reality he faced five days a week as the sun came up. Patients got the weekends off. Probably because the therapists got the weekend off. Play time all day Saturday. TV all day Saturday, except nap time. Discoveries to make. Adventures to experience. From the flat of the back. Or the bottom of the butt. Or crutched. The evil viri did not — could not — destroy the joy for most of the patients at Crippled Children's Hospital.

No matter how gimped up they were, the kids invented, reinvented and experienced over and over the pleasures of childhood. The sheer delight of *being* children. The evil viri could not take away the wonderland that filled those wards. Would that the same were true for rehabilitation afterlife.

Crippled Children's Hospital was a charity hospital. The fact that nobody had to pay if their families couldn't afford it saved a lot of lives during the years of the consumptive polio experience. Being a charity hospital meant a lot of other benefits for the patients. Organizations and people looking to do good works or looking to be thought of as doing good works showered offers of largesse upon the administrative offices.

In addition to the visits by movie and television stars there were also gifts at Christmas and other holiday times. The Easter bunny always made an appearance for all the children with lots and lots of goodies coming out of his basket. Halloween was filled with treats from folks who figured that that gesture bought them a couple of feet forward toward the pearly gates and a hair more protection from the fiery furnaces fueling hell's own reward for folks who didn't take care of crippled children.

There were a lot of invitations for activities for the kids who could leave the hospital for a couple of hours. Free tickets and transportation to the circus. A real treat — not like the scams proliferating today in which telephone boiler rooms beseech individuals and businesses to donate money to send crippled children to the circus and wind up pocketing seventy to ninety percent themselves. Where they'll sell ten thousand tickets for maximum seating of one thousand. They purport to be representing a local civic organization which, in fact, colluded in the fraud, accepting a few bucks as "inducements" to go along. And, the company who hires the telephone solicitors, owns the circus as well.

Once upon a time, when hearts were less larcenous, in nineteen-fifty-one, generous strangers came out of the night to usher a dozen mobile patients from Crippled Children's Hospital to a big stadium downtown where the city high school football championship was to be played. The friendly strangers finally got all the kids into the cars and limousines and station wagons and across town to the game. Front row seats for everybody. Right there on the sidelines by the home team's bench.

The Kid had never been to a football game. The Kid had never seen a football game. The Kid had never been around anyone who even talked about football.

The Kid was wrapped in a cocoon of blankets on the stretcher where he could see something. Actually, what he could see was a whole lot of ribcages. The stretcher was just over waist-high to the players. The game was an eye-level panorama that seemed to stretch distortedly forever before it disappeared into the black hole of the bleachers on the other side of the field.

He had no idea of what the hell was going on, but, whatever, it was fun to watch. Some guys stooping down digging a fist in the grass, then charging at each other like that bull in Paris used to charge Jacky and he, except they were running toward each other.

The air was charged with excitement. The Kid could feel it in every fiber of his being.

His stretcher was only a couple of feet from the waterbucket. One of the players coming off the field tossed his helmet under the bench, grabbed a towel, vigorously rubbed his face and hair and walked over to the waterbucket for a cool drink.

"Hey!" He grinned at the Kid. "Save your hey, you may have a cow some day!" Retorted the Kid. The player, who looked like he was as big as a cow himself, grinned. The Kid turned to one of his friends. "I guess I told him, didn't I."

Because Crippled Children's was a rehabilitation hospital, visiting hours were limited to once a week. On Sundays from two til four. Visitors every day would have made a mess of the treatment schedule, not mention playing havoc with the nerves of the help. Imagine a visiting parent's reaction when her dear, dear child screams in pain at the top of their lungs from the steaming hot packs Miss Bean slapped on their frail, defenseless body. Miss Bean would have a hard time straightening out her nose and growing her hair back. Wouldn't mean a damn whether it was good for them or not.

So every Sunday the aides helped all the patients spiff up in preparation for visiting hours. Typically, more than half the children had visitors from home. Mostly parents; sometimes aunts, uncles, even neighbors. No kids under sixteen were allowed.

Kids who'd lost the fight with the evil viri, or who kept fighting long enough, were sent to Crippled Adults' Hospital whose grounds adjoined the backyard of Crippled Children's Hospital. The Kid had heard the patients there were allowed visitors more frequently than once a week.

Crippled Children's did make exceptions to the Sunday only visitors rule. The Kid, for example, could not remember anyone visiting him during his entire stay at Crippled Children's Hospital in nineteen-fifty-one. He thinks perhaps he forgot someone. Surely, someone visited him during the week, taking advantage of the hospital's exception to its visiting rule. The Kid felt awfully lonesome whenever he tried to remember the truth-in-visiting-act of his first stay in Crippled Children's Hospital. Sadness is the only truth he can conjure here.

He can remember being scared that dad would try to visit him. Horror stories from Uncle Sam and grandmother about dad haunted him for years afterward. They had reconstructed him into a monster who would, if he came at all, burst through the front door of the hospital, stomp back into the ward, grab the Kid and walk away with him, carrying him to a life of unspeakable neglect.

Dad never came.

Meantime the Kid continued his trek down the road to rehabilitation. "We're going to teach you to act so normal that nobody'll ever know you had polio, boy. Here's what you've got to do: work. Work til you drop. Don't be easy on yourself, boy. That's a sign of weakness. If you're going to beat this thing and ever make anything out of yourself, you've got to work til it hurts and then keep on working."

The Kid followed this advice from doctors and therapists and discovered, thirty-some years later, they'd sentenced him to early terminal exhaustion. Their advice caused him to wear his body out by the time he was forty. When the world of practicing medicine finally accepted the reality of the late effects of polio in the late eighties, they advised post-polio people to slow down, to rest whenever they got tired.

BUT NOBODY KNEW WHAT TIRED WAS BE-CAUSE THE WHOLE GODDAMN MEDICAL ESTAB-LISHMENT HAD PERSUADED THEM TO IGNORE TIRED FOR SO LONG THE ONLY THING THEY KNEW WAS COMPLETE EXHAUSTION.

All the early warning systems had been short-circuited. In his later years the Kid would never again trust anyone with a degree in medicine.

Most of the patients of Crippled Children's Hospital were guinea pigs. Their families didn't have to pay for their rehabilitation. That was taken care of by Shelby County, the Kiwanis Clubs of West Tennessee and the March of Dimes. They paid in other ways. Every week a team of doctors marched through the wards raping and pillaging.

Doctor Ingram was, as far as the Kid knew, in charge of his treatment. Doctor Ingram was a stocky little man in a white coat who looked a whole lot like E. G. Robinson, the gangster actor. He'd smile and sometimes say hi before launching into his teaching mode.

"This patient is seven years old. Poliomyelitis. Atrophy of right leg, abdomen, back, and, less severely, in

127

the arms and left leg. Severe scoliosis, fifty-three degrees. Which has been worsening since his admission here in spite of the use of several supportive appliances, specifically a soft corset and a bed board. Patient will probably require surgical correction, although not at this time. Take his shirt off, nurse" — the doctor always took one of the *real* nurses along with them on their rounds — "and roll him over. Let's have a look-see."

"You" — he pointed to one of the student doctors — "show me with your finger the scoliosis on this patient. Yes, except you missed this section. Good! Any questions? You're doing fine, Kid. See you next week. Are they treating you okay?"

Every week there was a sideshow called doctor's rounds. Every week the freaks were the patients; the gawkers were the student doctors. Except for the weeks when visiting doctors from other areas of the country or other countries came with Doctor Ingram to see if they could learn something new about dealing with the devastation of the evil viri. They weren't any different from the students, however, it was still "get 'em naked, punch and pummel and pull and stretch and remould."

The medical community's insensitivity to the emotional needs of patients was never more apparent than in Crippled Children's Hospital. Not only did Doctor Ingram and others of his ilk give the orders which would too soon wear the tortured bodies out physically, they ignored the problems of isolation and emotional injury and turned back into the general population hundreds of thousands of kids who would never, who COULD NEVER be "normal" again. Rehab ignored almost every aspect of need except the pain wracked physical remedies. And the kids paid for it forever.

Separation. Abandonment. Anxiety.

Pathological distrust of both authority figures and those who purported to love.

In the early months of nineteen-fifty-one, the Kid was being heated and pummeled and churned into a semi-walking creature. From what he could learn from Doctor Ingram's passes by with the student doctors and what the Kid could feel himself when he tried to make routine gestures or movements which had become impossible, the Kid realized the evil viri had left his body pretty screwed up.

The scoliosis continued to deteriorate when the Kid was able to stand to begin his way back to walking. A steel-staved corset was the prescriptive answer. The aide would spread the opened corset on the bed, roll him onto it so his spine fit between the two big staves in back and pull the ends together. Buckle and tighten and truss. "Don't ever sit up without that corset, Kid. We've got to stop the scoliosis or you're going to have an operation on your back where we'll have to put sheep bone in there to fuse it straight."

The Kid didn't always follow rules. He hadn't always followed rules for his entire life since he was old enough for mom to give instructions. He sat up in bed in the afternoon during nap time without his corset. He sat up in bed at night during playtime without his corset.

So they brought out the torture machine. "Okay Kid, since you won't follow orders, we're going to make sure you don't sit up without your corset." They called it a "board". What it was was a steel frame just a little bigger and longer than the Kid with an iron cage hinged at the top, above the Kid's head, with loops for arms and legs, which swung down to fasten between the Kid's legs.

Just below the crotch. Every night all night the Kid slept on the board. Never turning. Barely moving. And every afternoon for naptime.

Neither Doctor Ingram nor the aides would listen to his protestations and promises that he would never ever misbehave again if they'd only give him one more chance. "Please...Please...Please..." Occasionally an aide would release him from his cage if the supervisor was out of the building.

The cage was torturous. In appearance. In fact. The Kid hated it.

The sinister inquisitors insisted it was his own fault, that if he'd laid flat on his back, like they'd been telling him for months, he'd never have had to have it.

Why can't they just leave me alone and let me be in peace? Every time they think about me they do something else to hurt me. Just leave me alone. Leave me alone. Get away from me!

The Kid almost never voiced the resentment he felt, for he knew that would lead to more punishment, more pain and more misery.

Why is it always me? Why doesn't anyone else get this much punishment? Every time somebody who's grownup walks through that door to the ward it seems like they're looking for me to do something else that's going to hurt. Why me!

In time, the Kid could sit in wheelchairs and stand and begin to walk. But first he had to have new shoes. Special shoes. High tops. With reinforced arch supports.

After early morning hot packs the Kid now went to the therapy room, pushed in a wheelchair, to practice walking. On a gadget that looked like a treadmill. Except it didn't move. With handrails that could be adjusted for the individual height of a patient. "You're going to be using crutches, Kid, so you're going to have to learn to walk with them, starting now. Right hand forward on the rail while your left leg goes forward. Now left hand forward on the rail while your right leg goes forward. And again and again and again until you've memorized it and can do it without even thinking about it. Walk. Walk. Step. Step. No. No! Not like that. Right hand, left foot! Right hand. Right hand! There.

For weeks.

Then with crutches. First with a belt around his waist held by the therapist to save him if he started to fall. And a week or so later without the safety belt. Until he had it down pat. Right crutch, left foot. Right foot, left crutch.

Exercise and hot packs.

Sometimes there was a surcease. Back then movie and television actors liked to think they were doing their part for the anti-polio effort by visiting kids hit by the evil viri at bedside in hospitals. With a large entourage of reporters and photographers.

One afternoon just before the end of nap time a pretty woman swept through the ward with a bunch of people around her, treating her like she was some kind of queen. Beds were arranged in two rows each butting up to opposite walls with the head closest to the wall and the foot pointing to the center walkway. She started flouncing down the right side row, stopping at each bed and giving the patient a choice of a jigsaw puzzle or some other geegaw. And, of course, an opportunity to see her.

None of the patients knew who she was, only that she must be important for the whole hospital to stop for her visit. What the hell! It was no skin off the patients' back to skip a therapy session or a hot pack or some of that other misery they handed out in the name of healing. *Bring 'em on. I hope she stays til supper. Walk slow. No hurry. No hurry at all.*

The Kid's bed was the last she visited in the ward. She flounced demurely toward him. Dark short hair. Smile. *She does have a pretty smile. She looks like she might care. Look at the way she's looking at me like I'm somebody special. Isn't she pretty!* She was pretty, he had to admit that, but she sure wasn't "sexy", not like Annie Catherine or Linda Lou Hart or Dovey Cole were. She gave his seven year old libido a shiver, but she didn't give him that special wrenching feeling way down to the bottom of his belly. But, she was pretty. And the Kid was a sucker for a smile and attention from anybody. "And how are you today, Kid?" The name of each patient was taped to the foot of the bed so it wasn't truly miraculous that she came to him knowing his name. She leaned over and kissed him on the forehead, leaving a clear imprint of her lips. He was thrilled.

"My name's Mona. Here's a little something that I hope will help you remember me by. All I have left is a jigsaw puzzle. Is that alright?" "Mmmm Hmm." Someone handed her a box which she gently placed on the Kid's bed near his head. And here's an autographed picture of me just for you. You can tape this on your bed if you like." And swept out of the ward. The name on the picture was Mona Freeman.

Francis the Talking Mule showed up at the hospital one day. Francis the Talking Mule was just about the Kid's favorite character in all the movies he saw. He was not only smarter than all the grownup human beings in the movie, he was hilarious as he made asses of them.

Later on the Kid would liken the character to the puppet who was, in reality, the puppeteer. All the kids who could be moved gathered between the big front porch and the long driveway to see the star of so many of the movies they'd seen. Unlike the lady actor, they ALL knew who Francis was.

Strangely enough, though, his trainer couldn't persuade him to utter a word that day. He could make him sit in his (the trainer's) lap. He could coax him into dancing and counting (by pawing the pavement with his right front hoof) and laughing ("mule" laugh). Nowhere could he find a word. Still, just seeing him was a big treat.

Despite repeated promises by the short man who taught Sunday School, Jesus never did come around to save or heal or entertain the kids. Jesus never did show up although a gang of patients used to sit up nights waiting for Him to come down and make whatever it was that had been visited upon them go away. He didn't. It didn't.

Whatever torture the medicos had put the Kid through must have accomplished something beyond satisfying the individual therapists' deep-rooted hunger for sadistic satisfaction because he *was* walking again. Very slowly. With crutches. Right crutch forward. Left crutch forward. Right leg forward. Slowly but slowly the Kid could walk the length of the corridor. He could walk all the way from the ward to the auditorium. To the therapy room. And back.

Then one day Doctor Ingram pronounced the Kid fit to go. "I might be seeing you back here in a few years, Kid. If your scoliosis fails to stabilize. If your back keeps getting more and more crooked. But right now there's nothing else we can do. The physical therapist will give you some exercises that you must do every day. You'll

133

need to come back to Memphis for check-ups every few months. Wear your corset all the time when you're not lying down. Don't try to walk without those special shoes, because you need extra support now. Always use your crutches when you walk.

The thought of going home rang sweetly through the Kid's head on that morning in the spring of nineteen-fifty-one. There were, however, three, maybe four, klaxon horns doing their damnedest to warn the Kid of impending danger. The Kid knew the choices. He had to leave the hospital because they said he had to go. That left Uncle Sam's farm out by Mansfield. That was the choice. Circle one.

The next day Uncle Sam made an appearance at the door.

Mrs. Robinson walked up to Uncle Sam. "Are you the boy's father?" "No, I'm his uncle but I'm his guardian." "So you'll be responsible for him when he gets home?" "Yes ma'am." "Okay, there are some exercises and other instructions that I need to give you before you leave. Lie down, Kid, let's demonstrate:

> —lying flat on his stomach with legs extended, have him raise his head and shoulders as far up from the floor or bed as possible, ten times three times a day.

If you can, you should put a board between the mattress and springs of his bed.

> —lying on his left side, he needs to raise his right leg as high as he can and hold it for a count of two. Then slowly lower it. Ten times three times a day.

—right side, Kid, raise your left leg. Higher. Higher. Now hold it for a count of two. And lower it, slowly. Ten times three times a day.

—sit, with legs stretched out. Without bending your knees put your nose between your knees. If he has trouble with this somebody should hold his knees down.

This is all very important to stretch his muscles as much as possible back to the shape they were in before he contracted polio.

—lie flat on your back. Lift your left leg. Slowly. As high as you can. Hold for two counts. Slowly lower it back. Ten times three times a day.

—and your right leg. The same routine. And slowly back to the bed.

Now you'll notice he can't lift his right leg off the bed at all. This is where he'll need help every time until the muscle tone returns. [It never did.] While he is trying as hard as he can to lift the leg, you lift it by the foot just like the other leg. Hold for a count of two, always making sure that he is really trying and not letting you do all the work. He will also need to continue taking naps in the afternoon. At least two hours after lunch."

"Now if you'll come with me to the office the Kid can say his goodbyes." The Kid joyfully bade his friends farewell. With a smirk. He had beaten them home. He had won the race. He was first. But when it came time to say goodbye to the adults he choked up. And didn't know why he felt like crying when Miss Bean hugged him. And the occupational therapists, the physical therapist, Miss Graves and even the big boss. Seemed to him that he should have been happier. Instead it was terribly depressing.

Miss Bean packed up the Kid's comic books and the real watch which he had taken apart and couldn't get back together. And the Kid was outta there.

Uncle Sam walked with him out the front door and lifted the frail body into the cab of the Dodge. "Ready?" "Yessir." "Let's go!" And away they went. Stopping only for gas, a hamburger with pickles, onions and mustard, and a coke.

It was invigorating to be in the wide open air again, to be able to smell the diesel fumes of Trailways busses which bespoke of untold adventures on the highway.

Problem was he didn't feel free as the wind. As he was riding shotgun in the psychedelic Dodge pickup that day, the Kid didn't feel like the carefree child he had been when Jacky and he used to run like the wind to escape the butcher knife gang or even when Joel and he used to run and jump and chase clouds and shadows all over the Mansfield farm.

As he huddled next to the passenger door peering longingly through the mottled glass he could feel the shackles the evil viri had locked his body inside. He could feel the steel-staved corset that squeezed his body tightly under the new shirt Aunt Naomi had sewn. His mind hated everything about it and what it meant to him, not being able to walk or run or play like he always used to. No matter that it made him stand taller and sit straighter and that they said it just might stave off the surgeon's knife for a few years. And his feet. Bound in the brand new shoes they'd given him to support his feet properly so he could walk. They'd told him that his feet would not be strong enough to go barefoot, probably never again. Ever. And the crutches.

The always hated, ever-present crutches.

Back in the Bosom

Home again! Springtime in Mansfield, Tennessee. The green and white house sat like a decoration on top of a cake baked for the Kid's homecoming. A summer breeze rustled the leaves on the big trees in a sparsely grassed yard. The shadow of clouds rolled across the roof and over the house. The barn and fields beyond. And the railroad in the distant.

The Dodge pickup threw up a rooster-tail of dust for a quarter of a mile back down the curvy gravel road before it braked ten feet short of the front stoop.

In a world where words had lost most of their impact the Kid was filled with mixed emotions. He was thrilled to be getting out of the confines of the hospital and into some wide open spaces where he and Joel could play to their hearts content. But he was distressed at the prospect of being the pupil in more of Uncle Sam's patented disciplinary classes. The past months had not diminished the memory of those sessions of passion and pain.

He liked Uncle Sam. He really did. Uncle Sam and he got along fine most of the time, especially since the attack of the evil viri. But when Uncle Sam hardened his eyes in anger or disagreement the Kid cringed and prayed for mercy from God, just in case. Only after those eyes softened could the Kid breathe again. The hospital and maybe the terrible shape the evil viri had made of his body were, the Kid fervently hoped, a defense against those sessions.

What really happened was that Uncle Sam got the best of both worlds. He didn't beat the Kid bloody after

138

polio, but he increased the passionate diatribes. Even though the worst of actual physical abuse was chased away forever by the evil viri, face-slapping apparently was not included in the lexicon of handicapper abuse. The Kid had been pummeled so many times in the past that any time Uncle Sam so much as raised his voice he might as well have been swinging that blood-seeking belt because that's what it would feel like to the Kid. Forever more.

Aunt Naomi stood there at the top of the front porch steps, her hands resting on her hips. She had an interesting figure. Long curly hair. Eyes that stuck out just enough to be sexy, like Annie Catherine's. The Kid couldn't remember the size of her bosoms but he remembered everything tapering down to this tiny waist then flaring out again into normal sized hips and a belly that was attractively Rubenesque. She was pretty, the Kid thought.

She came down the steps in her patterned housedress and walked over to the passenger side of the truck, opened the door, reached in and gave the Kid a big hug. "Welcome home mister. We've missed you around here. It's been too quiet without you. Now maybe it'll liven up. Hope so, anyway."

The Kid took his first steps as a gimp on the farm as Joel ran up from behind for a front row seat.

"Hi." The Kid to Joel.

"Howdy." Joel to the Kid.

All the attention the Kid got must have upset Joel at some level. That could explain Joel blaming the Kid later on for mischief he himself had made. There had been some of that before the evil viri. It got much worse before the Kid finally yelled calf rope.

"You and Joel have your old room back. And there's a slop jar right here by the bed in case you need to go to the bathroom at night. I don't want any peeing on the floor."

"Okay, lie down. Time for your exercises." Uncle Sam was not a born physical therapist. Nor was he much better after months of practice. Whenever he lent a hand it was more like he was hitching up the mule to a plow on a day when he'd rather be pitching shit than plowing fields but would have been well satisfied to do neither. There wasn't much gentle about him physically, except when he was dealing with Aunt Naomi and Joel.

It didn't appear to be deliberate with the Kid, however, just a knee-jerk-barely-contained savagery against the progeny of the wild beast who'd dared tempt his wife in a strange bed. Or car. Or bush. But, now, around Aunt Naomi he minded his manners or she'd give him a sample of that acid attack tongue she hung onto for emergencies. Nossir that lady wore the britches in the family and Uncle Sam never forgot that except when he ran off to drink himself silly in town.

The very next morning after he got home, Uncle Sam had gone to the fields immediately after breakfast. A few minutes later the school bus pulled up to the house, right into the yard. Aunt Naomi walked out onto the porch, the Kid right behind her.

Am I going to school? Nobody told me. Wow! If the bus came all the way over here I must be going to school. It's a surprise is what it is! Aunt Naomi was going to surprise me!

140

"Figured the Kid could use a hand, so I drove up here to pick him up." "Oh, Raleigh, thank you, but he ain't strong enough to go to school. He has to stay home, at least for the rest of this year. But it's real kind of you to do this. Thank you." *I knew it was too much to hope for. I should have known they'd make me stay home to take my nap and do my exercises.*

Disappointment.

What happened was the Kid got a homebound teacher, Miz Richardson, who drove out to the house two or three times a week to hand out assignments, pick up assignments and give him gentle instructions to sugar the medicine. He liked her. A lot. Later she would be Ronald's first grade teacher, which would make him jealous because he felt like she belonged to him. And understandably so because he'd always dealt with her on a one-on-one basis. Never had had to share her with other kids or anyone else.

He liked doing homework.

He didn't like doing his exercises and taking his naps but Aunt Naomi wasn't about to let him slack there. Nosirree. That woman was there on time every time with a plan and a tongue you dasn't call down upon yourself.

After dinner at noontime she'd take off his corset, make him take off his shoes and bed him down for his two hour nap. Now what seven year old is going to sleep for two hours every afternoon when the rest of the whole wide world is out yonder having fun? Joel didn't have to take a nap. He'd get up from the table and make a dash outside. Uncle Sam would go back to the fields. But, no, the Kid had to go to bed. Aunt Naomi didn't exactly nap, but she'd sit in a rocking chair in the living room letting the refrains of country music relax her while the Kid was supposedly sleeping.

The Kid loved music. He'd pick up anything handy as he lay on Joel's and his bed and shake it like a tambourine or hit it against the heel of his hand like musical spoons, keeping time to the music. It was fun and kept him awake and gave him something to do.

Until the afternoon Aunt Naomi walked in and demanded, "What's that noise I've been hearing all afternoon? Listen to me, Kid. Every time a song started playing on the radio I heard a sound like a rattle or something. I know you've got something. Now give it to me." The Kid reluctantly handed it over. "You've been intentionally staying awake while you're supposed to be sleeping. For that I'm going to throw it away and I'm going to add a half hour onto your naptime today. Now go to sleep. The sooner you do the sooner you can get up."

The evil viri had blasted a hole the size of west Tennessee in the Kid's relationship with Joel. Before last November they had run and played and fought and rough-housed from the time they got up until suppertime except when the Kid had to work. The difference now was night and day. No more rough-housing. Orders from headquarters. No running. No playing except when the Kid was sitting. No swinging from the crutches which was the only way the Kid could pick up a little speed. No this. No that.

What Joel heard was that the Kid was off limits because he was so fragile he might break something if they played together. So he became an only child again and went off to amuse himself most of the day. About the only time they had together anymore was reading some of the Kid's comic books — by now the pile had grown to more than three feet high — or when they were forced together for something boring like eating or church or visiting.

The Kid's choice of playmates had pretty much dwindled down to his pick of the pigs or the chickens.

The Kid finished the second grade and started the third grade with his homebound teacher presented through the good graces of the Henry County Board of Education. His grades were As and Bs, a helluva sight better than they had been a year earlier when readin' and writin' and 'rithmetic had been just about the last things on his mind, down there with going to church and behaving like the model child Uncle Sam insisted he be. He now became a veritable bookworm, a creature of study habits.

As the newness of his crippledom wore off Uncle Sam and Aunt Naomi turned the microscope way down. The Kid could wander at will through the yard and go down behind the barn and bring the cows home of a night. He could play with Joel as long as he didn't try to run. Aunt Naomi would run out of the kitchen like an insane Jesus when she saw him picking up a little speed to keep up with or try to outrun Joel.

Manners. The Kid did learn his manners as a member of the dysfunctional family. Yes ma'am. Nossir. May I please? Wait til someone offers you something; don't grab. Don't ever take the last of food from a bowl on the table. That's real close to a hanging offense. And the pounding and vicious words ingrained a deep reticence within him to confront anyone about anything forevermore.

On Easter Sunday the whole Sutton clan gathered at grandmother's house for the Easter egg hunt. Some of the aunts and uncles would go round hiding the dyed boiled eggs in bushes, forks of trees, flowerbeds, tall grass, loose boards and any other hiding place they could find. Then they let the kids loose. Finders keepers. The usual crowd was Larry and Johnny (Aunt Margaret), Billy and Barbara (Uncle J), Joel (Uncle Sam), Peggy, Jacky, the Kid and Ronald (mom). The Kid was afraid to get very excited about the great Easter egg hunt of nineteen-fifty-one. He was sure one or both of the heads of household of the extended family would cut him off at the pass with a kick in the emotional ass. He was wrong.

They let him crutch his way to half a dozen hiding places. With a little help from his cousins, which he chose to ignore. Still, when Larry ran up and said, "there's one over there," and pointed as he slowed down but made like he was speeding up and let the Kid get there just a hair ahead of him to grab the prize, in retrospect it could be said with some measure of confidence that his pursuit of the egg was not entirely independent. What it did was make him happy as a pig in shit. The Kid got a belly ache from eating all the eggs he found. Most of the kids did.

Family gatherings were great pepper-uppers for the Kid. Leaving them to go back to Mansfield left a pit the size of Rhode Island in his belly, aching and feeling like he'd felt when everybody left him in Isolation Hospital to go back home to Henry County.

If it hadn't been for his fear of the wrath and retribution, the summer of nineteen-fifty-one would have been wonderful. Linda Ann had been born in July. Joel was six. He and the Kid got matching straw hats with sweatbands inside to soak up the sweat to cool you off.

Exercise three times a day under the supervision of Aunt Naomi. A two hour nap every afternoon under the eagle eye of Aunt Naomi. When he wasn't doing his exercises or resting and when Joel wasn't too antsy, the Kid and Joel played a lot of marbles that summer. In direct contradiction of orders the Kid insisted they play "for keeps", that is, whoever won an opponent's marble got to keep the marble forever. Both aunt and uncle had ruled that out because Joel was two years younger and playing keeps would be unfair to him. The Kid, however, wasn't real particular about the morality of the conduct required to add to his jar of marbles.

Two or three times Uncle Sam would get up early — way before daylight — to milk the cows and do the morning chores before tossing the Kid into the Dodge pickup and trucking on down to Memphis for checkups at the Shelby County Health Clinic stuck in a little nook by the side of Baptist Hospital.

First thing is the x-ray guy would take x-rays of the Kid's scoliosis. Then Uncle Sam and the Kid would go back to the waiting room for two or three hours. For however long it took for the Kid's name to be called. He'd then go to one of the tiny dressing rooms separating the waiting room from the examination area, take off his clothes and put on a hospital gown and underwear that looked more like a surgical mask you'd tie between your legs, and wait until someone led him into an examination room where he'd wait until someone came by to examine him. Sometimes that someone was Doctor Ingram; sometimes that someone was a student doctor.

This was very good practice for student doctors. They practiced for years on the post-polio people who flooded their doorways.

145

Uncle Sam would report back to Henry County. "He's doing okay. You should see how pitiful some of the other kids they bring in there are. There's no reason to feel sorry for him. At least he can walk with crutches. Some of them can't even sit up, much less stand."

Aside from the terse conversation he always had with the x-ray guy, the Kid enjoyed the sojourn to Memphis. Especially the hamburger stop at a greasy spoon along U.S. 79. Uncle Sam stopped at a number of different restaurants along the way but the hamburgers always tasted the same. Something along the lines of a White Castle gut bomb except a helluva lot better. The Kid loved those hamburgers all to pieces and would, later, rue the simple times when a wonderful greasy hamburger tasted like a wonderful greasy hamburger.

The Sam Sutton household didn't have an indoor toilet. There was a two-holer out back of the house. A closet built downwind from the manse. Wiping with the pages from a Sears and Roebuck mail order catalog. A thick catalog would last months before they got down to used newsprint and paper bags. They never used corncobs. The Kid was happy with the toileting arrangement. After all, except for the few months in the hospital he didn't know anything else. And that experience dulled quickly.

One sunny morning during the summer of fifty-one he walked his four-point walk down to the john, unbuckled the straps to his overalls, pushed his pants down and sat on the right hole to "do his business". As he sat there concentrating on the business at hand, feeling the relief that only a bowel movement can bring, he heard a soft rustling noise. And thought nothing more of it. Until he heard it again. Seemingly closer. And looked over his left shoulder to see what appeared to be movement on

146

the wall behind him. He looked closer. He saw a brightly colored snake crawling down one of the cracks in the back wall toward his butt!

As if the Lord God Almighty hisself had cured him, the Kid ran from that place.

Without benefit of crutches.

Without benefit of pulling his overalls up above his ankles.

Without any benefit except the horror that that legless beast was going to bite his ass if he didn't get out of there. Right now!

Of course, as with much spiritual healing, when the post-hypnotic suggestion wears off the healing disappears. Somewhere in the grass eight to ten feet from the privy the Kid's healing evaporated. He fell. Terrified.

Until Aunt Naomi heard his hysterical blathering and came out to see what the fuss was all about, and, responding to his flailing gesticulations, approached the outhouse. "It's not there now, Kid. I don't see a sign of a snake. You don't have to worry. It's gone. Besides it was probably just a chicken snake. It wouldn't have hurt you. Matter of fact it was prob'ly as scared of you as you were of it."

She reached into the privy and brought his crutches out. Then helped him to his feet and with his overalls after she'd brought him the catalog to finish wiping himself with — no amount of persuasion would get him back onto that toilet — and guided him back to the big house.

The Kid would never again for the rest of his life be able to look at an outside toilet without recoiling in

147

fear. And the times he actually used one, over the rest of his life, he did so out of absolute necessity and every time could feel that snake crawling down the wall behind him and raising its head to get a better angle of his ass. Shit or die. That was the question.

One day a Paris doctor said the Kid better get his tonsils taken out, else he was gonna die, because "they were poisoning his system." And so it was that Uncle Sam and Aunt Naomi took him up to the clinic. The next morning somebody put a hospital gown on him, placed him on a stretcher and pushed him into the operating room and transferred him to the operating table. He was so sorely afraid that he couldn't even pee his pants.

As he lay quaking someone stuck a gauze mask on his face and looked into his eyes. "Hi, I'm Doctor Sumthin-or-other. Are we a mite scared this morning?" "Yessir." "Well, don't worry too much, we'll make you comfortable and this'll all be over before you know it. I'm going to put some ether on your mask. It's going to make you very sleepy. Don't fight it. When you feel like going to sleep, go to sleep and when you wake up you'll be back in your room good as new without those old tonsils that are making you sick. Have you got a girlfriend?" "Yessir." "What's her name?" "Dovey." "Is she pretty?" "Yessir." "Have you told her yet?" "Nossir."

And that's the last the Kid remembered until he woke up a couple of hours later, puking. Sicker'n a dog. From the ether. With a sore throat. Spitting blood. With a roomful of company: Uncle Sam, Aunt Naomi, grandmother, Peggy. Peggy brought him some ice cream which also made him sick until the ether wore off.

It was nice, though, having all that attention and people bringing him presents. The Kid just about purred when somebody petted him.

He later thought it was strange that there were no memories of Jacky. At the big Christmas doings during his furlough from Isolation Hospital. After his tonsils were pulled. They'd been closer than glue at the loghouse and now, in the Kid's memory banks, Jacky seemed to have disappeared. It was Peggy he remembered as the caring sibling who showed up with a wallet for Christmas and ice cream for the sore throat. Where was Jacky? And Ronald? Was it a conveniently faulty memory and, if so, why?

There were problems that could not be overcome. The Kid still wet the bed at night. Which was interesting in that he hadn't wet the bed in the hospital. And the Kid still had the attitude of a troubled eight year old which seemed never to work in that setting.

Uncle Sam died of some kind of dread cancer in the mid-sixties. The Kid didn't go to the funeral. Ironically, Uncle Sam was living with grandmother when he died. In a little mobile home down by the pasture in front of Uncle J's and Aunt Lillian's house on Mansfield Road. A long time later the Kid got to thinking that he wasn't as bad as he acted. Uncle Sam had lots of worries about finances, his marriage, his booze habit, jealousy of the success of many of his siblings. He would understand that while he was often the target of Uncle Sam's rage he was not the cause of it, only the igniter. Being a brat didn't help. Being Connie Moody's son certainly didn't help.

The unanswered sixty-four dollar question is why in hell no one in the family saw what was happening to the boy and step in to help!

Grandmother always said, "Sam Sutton is as hard working as any boy of mine. He can't help it what he does. He got messed up by that ole' war and he ain't been no good since." The tears begin to flow down her cheeks at this point. "He was just as good as they git. I raised him. I know how he was. Naomi would never give him credit for nothing. I know he's done wrong but she could give him some support. She could help him to make it. That's why they had to leave the farm. Naomi wasn't about to go out of her way to help him, even if it meant they'd have to leave. I'll tell you one thing about Naomi; she ain't goin' do a lick of work 'less she's got to. Not one lick."

Just a matter of degrees of temperament. Say he hadn't gone to war, he'd probably would have had only half as many shit fits over half as many "situations" and beaten the Kid half as many licks half as many times. Which would have left the Kid black and blue and bleeding half as many times.

But almost certainly just as fucked up.

Still, it's better to understand those things.

Isn't it?

The Kid ran away from home again. In a sense. All he remembers is being at grandmother's house in Paris. He might have told a cousin he didn't want to live there anymore and the cousin probably conveyed the message to an adult who more than likely told grandmother who told Uncle Sam who'd been calmed down enough by Aunt Naomi to actually talk about it in the absence of a boiling rage. "Don't you want to live with us anymore, Kid?" Aunt Naomi asked. "No ma'am." "Why?" Silence. "Why, Kid?" Silence. "Don't you have a reason? Can't you even give us a reason?"

"I don't want to get the cows anymore." The Kid was too scared to tell the truth. How can an eight year old child tell an adult who's abusing him the reason he wants to leave is because of the abuse. The Kid remembers feeling relief that the parting conversation didn't explode into violence.

"Okay, if you're sure. It's your decision, Kid. You can come live with your grandmother. We've done all we can. We've treated you like a son but if you wanna go, there's no sense in us trying to hold on to you."

Somehow, in the middle of the third grade, the Kid was able to move from Mansfield to Paris with his important parts intact.

Grandmother was a kvetcher. Every single one of the Kid's siblings wound up with lots of resentment against her because she often couldn't see beyond the end of her nose.

The Kid somehow remembered not so much about her bitching, but how she had helped. In the long run grandmother was no more than a gnat. She only spanked the Kid for wetting the bed. He was used to that.

City Life

West Paris was the poor side of town. West Paris was the place of peasantry. Comfortable chunky old ladies side by side with real skinny old ladies, house dresses covered with aprons working in their gardens and flower gardens and gossiping up and down the street. From porch to porch. Yard to yard. Mostly a couple of notches above poor white trash in the social pecking order of northwest Tennessee.

West Paris was where grandmother and granddaddy moved to when they left the Moody clan back at the Hancock place. To a neighborhood called Rorie Addition. Rorie was the guy who had made a lot of money putting up houses in the area. Lower-middle class houses. Mixed in with some middle-middle class houses. With a sprinkling of upper-lower class and even some middle-lower class housing here and there.

Grandmother's house was one of those "fixer-uppers". Granddaddy had hoped to put some money in the bank for the retirement that was supposed to have come from work in Detroit, but didn't. Four big rooms built in crackerbox fashion: living room on the northeast side; kitchen to the northwest; granddaddy and grandmother's bedroom to the southwest and the spare bedroom to the southeast, the bedroom the Moody clan would march through.

There were also two small rooms at the back of the house. One, just off the master bedroom would eventually be divided in half becoming the indoor bathroom and the other half the junk room. The second, back of the kitchen, would be Peggy's bedroom until the day she ran off to Corinth, Mississippi and married Joe Frankie Smith at the age of fifteen.

The roof was corrugated tin, except for Peggy's bedroom which had tarpaper covering it. The house was built on the side of a gently sloping hill that ran from Miz Bollus' house to an empty field. The south side sat on the ground. The north side rose between four and five feet off the ground. The front porch ran the width of the house. There was a rickety back porch which grandmother used for the likes of washing and drying fruit for fried pies.

She had an old Kenmore wringer washer that would shake what few nails were left in the planking looser every time it went through the bouncy cycle. The water came from a garden hose hooked up to the "hydrant" which is what they called the outdoor spigot.

First they filled the washing machine for the really big job of getting the dirt and grime out. And then the washtub which she used for rinsing. There was a double roller on a pivoting arm above the washer for wringing out the clothes. I guess that's why they called them wringer washers. Although it wasn't a wringer at all. It was really more of a squeezer. Grandmother fed the clothes one piece at a time, careful of fingers, through the moving rollers which squeezed most of the moisture out, probably as much to save water as to start the drying process. Sometimes something big, like a hand or arm would jam up the wringer and she'd have to slam the emergency release bar near the top, popping the rollers apart so they wouldn't separate the offending arm from its body or drag the rest of the body through.

Once the clothes were properly rinsed and safely squeezed through the wringer, they'd go on the clothes-lines, of which there were two: a single line from the back porch to the chicken pen out back and a double line running under the apple tree on the north side of the house from the front porch almost to the flower garden.

Monday was washday. Between six and seven to make sure nobody was going to sleep all day if she had to break her back over a hot washtub. Grandmother made a big to do over washday. It seemed to give essence to her martyrdom.

Grandmother was a wonderful martyr. And she was so proud of being a martyr that she'd tell anybody who listened for more than a minute at least one reason why she qualified for the lifetime achievement award for martyrdom.

At the back of the house there had once been a well on the porch, before city water came, which was attested to by a reddish-brown tile sticking a foot or so above the porch floor. There was a cistern at the end of the back porch which at one time caught and saved rain-water for household use. Granddaddy had nailed a plank cover over it. Grandmother planted four o'clocks and other flowers around it to make it beautiful.

Indoor plumbing was not much in vogue in Paris, Tennessee, in the early fifties. There was an outdoor toilet back of the flower garden. A single sitter. Granddaddy dug a big-ass hole that must have been four and a half feet deep and six feet long. He dug it so well that the john didn't have to be moved again before indoor plumbing came to 314 Hooper Street. And to add even more sophistication to body elimination someone had built a rose-bush lined pathway from the back porch to the outhouse.

Truth to tell, the house was pretty rundown before granddaddy got to work. He put on a new roof and new siding. He put in a new front porch and separated the staves in the little fence that ran its length so your legs could catch some of the breeze of a summer's day when temperatures were known to climb over the one-hundred degree mark regularly. Granddaddy was a good carpenter, as far as the Kid was concerned. But the house in Rorie Addition, no matter what he did to it, looked about like what you would expect to see in a house in Rorie Addition. About like you'd expect to see in a house on a dirt farm in Henry County. Falling in on itself as he got too sick to work on anything anymore.

And then he died. The Kid was living there when granddaddy died. It was springtime nineteen-fifty-two when the Kid packed up his clothes and went to live at grandmother's. Somebody had appropriated a hospital bed that could be cranked up, head and foot, for granddaddy's comfort. That was in the living room along with his special chair. The Kid used to agonize over not having a memory of what granddaddy did to pass the time during those months between his heart attack and the tap tapping of the grim reaper's scythe. Did he read? Listen to the radio? Or did he die of terminal boredom?

Ronald remembered the night granddaddy died. "He ate supper in the kitchen with the rest of us, went into the living room, sat down in his chair, and died."

The Kid remembered only that his body was in a casket in the living room. Or was it in the front bedroom? He remembered seeing him lying there with his hands crossed, looking like his face was moulded out of wax or something.

So much for the accuracy of history. But the whole of the family does agree that granddaddy did in fact die one day. What was left of granddaddy was an eight-by-ten black and white picture placed on the mantel, sitting on a quilt, the sleeves of his white shirt rolled up to mid-bicep. He looked at peace with the world, away from the uproar minding his own business and reveling in the quietude.

I don't know why they didn't split the kids up after granddaddy died but they didn't. Home there would never quite be the same again. There would never again be the calmative influence he had over the household in the maelstrom of grandmother's incessant complaints. All the kids missed him.

Life on Hooper Street was sweet for the Kid. As sweet as the pollen he used to suck out of honeysuckle blossoms. Not only did he not have to go get the cows anymore he didn't have to do jackshit except polish the furniture and the floors and sideboards around the linoleum rugs in the living room, front bedroom and kitchen. That's it.

Rumor was grandmother wasn't a great cook. Extensive efforts to ferret out positive comments about grandmother's cooking over a period of three decades has been totally hopeless. Not one compliment to grandmother the chef could be found — except the Kid, of course — and nobody paid much any attention to his tastes anyhow. It is, however, the Kid's belief that the Moody kids kinda liked what she put before them on that old tin dining table. After the stuff they'd been fed by dad after mom died just about anything was good eatin'. Whatever way she fixed food was the right way — with the possible exception of Peggy's opinion. What's a few burnt crusts and tough biscuits among siblings compared to no food at all.

For as long as he would live, the Kid believed the only good biscuits were flat and tough as leather. And who ever makes decent toast anymore? Grandmother would butter one side of half a dozen pieces of white bread, put them in a baking pan and in the oven under the broiler until the butter melted and the crust browned or burned. Who said she couldn't cook.

It didn't take long for the Kid to learn to like the city. All those people. All that stuff going on. Life was 'bout as perfect as it could get. The family was together again.

Except for mom and dad. Except it didn't always seem like love and togetherness when grandmother went on one of her verbal rampages against the evils of the Moody father. Except how come it still felt so empty and lonesome when kinfolk went home on a Sunday afternoon? How come the Kid was always wishing he was going with 'em? Or that he was living with the Watsons or Uncle Nolan and Aunt Louise. How come that?

There was never an unhappy or dull moment at Aunt Louise's house when the Kid went visiting what with Linda and Fay and Johnny and Carol Ann. Aunt Louise was no pushover but she was loving, both vocally and physically. They'd go into Puryear every weekend for a movie in the tent by Rhodies or groceries or something. The Kid remembered somebody picking him up and standing him in the back of a flatbed truck so he could draw the name of a lucky lottery winner.

Johnny's room was upstairs. By invitation only. That was the big thrill of the trip; to be invited into the inner sanctum for a few minutes. The Kid wished he could be as smart as Johnny who was as close as the Kid would get to a role model. At the end of his stay the Kid would say goodbye to his cousins, Aunt Louise and Uncle Nolan, with a big lump in his throat and the wish he could have stayed out there with them for the rest of his life.

There were kids in the neighborhood and cousins who came by in a constant stream in the summertime to play hide-and-seek and kick-the-can. 'Course the Kid's orders were: "Donchu git out there with them kids. Don't try to run. Sit down on the porch and watch. It's for your own good, Kid. If ye git out there and try to run like them other kids yer goin' mess yerself up for the rest of your life. I know ye'd like to, but ye can't. At least ye can be around 'em."

Tommy Fox was his friend who bummed around with him. There was always some place to make a fort or ward off marauding Indians or to stake a claim and build a cabin. Unfortunately that somewhere was usually on the other side of the fence and grandmother forbade the Kid from leaving the yard. And he obeyed. When he could.

Life as a gimp had its off moments. It wasn't easy to sneak around so the Kid was always lobbying for a game site up the hill or in the back of the house or some other venue which was not constantly eyeballed by adults sittin' on him to sit on the ground and watch his world go by "for your own good." He had to exercise three times a day. He had to take a two hour nap. Every day.

Grandmother would occasionally untie the bow of her apron to give the Kid some breathing room. His particular favorite was to visit the Flinns who lived up the street. Mr. Flinn was a railroad worker. The Kid was the recipient of all Mr. Flinn's expired union pins. Mostly Mr. Flinn was at work. Railroad people were often gone for days at a time. It was a special treat for the Kid to spend an afternoon with Mrs. Flinn in the living room of that tiny house up the hill. Welcoming, like a warm hug. The Kid liked it a lot.

The one thing that didn't stop at grandmother's was the bedwetting. The Kid would wake up in the middle of the night in the bed he shared with Jacky with something warm spreading down his leg. He desperately wanted to quit. He had heard grandmother talking about Jacky and Peggy also being bedwetters so he didn't feel absolutely all alone, but he did feel absolutely frustrated because they were the only two people on the planet who would believe that he didn't do it on purpose.

On the mornings after he had wet the bed the night before, the Kid's dread of grandmother came close to that he'd held for Uncle Sam. "Now go out in the yard and get me a keen switch from the peach tree and bring it here." The Kid would break off a small branch from the tree, strip it clean of leaves and take it to grandmother who then commenced to infuse him with "peach tree tea." She'd hold one of his hands and switch him with the other. It didn't matter whether his legs were fucked up or not the Kid danced to run away from that stinging. Every lick was like being stung by a dozen wasps. To make him mend his ways and train his bladder to keep the bed dry all night. Perhaps there was in fact some Pavlovian value in the switching, for almost never did there occur a bedwetting the night immediately following a switching.

Miz Richardson came by two or three times a week to review the work the Kid was doing and to leave more assignments so he wouldn't get behind the kids in

159

regular class. He enjoyed that a lot, but he never thought of what he was doing as real school. To him it was pretend. She was pretending to be a teacher and he was pretending to be a student and he loved it, especially the part about pretending to study to see how well he could do even though it didn't count for anything. It was a neat game.

One of the first things grandmother did after the Kid came to live with her was to buy a desk. It was for everyone. She made that perfectly clear. But it was also for the Kid's school work. One of the pictures in the Paris newspaper around March of Dimes fundraising time was of the Kid standing in his bib overalls braced by his crutches at the corner of that desk. Pretty little country gimp bumpkin. Sparkling blue eyes. Dishwater brown hair. Charming smile. Bet he woulda drove the nine year old girls wild. Sure.

Between his own desire to show off and grandmother's demand that he get his "work" done, he spent a lot of hours at the desk.

One morning grandmother went up the street to gossip with one of the neighbors leaving the Kid alone in the house to do his work for Miz Richardson's next trip. He was in his usual study mode: shoulders hunched in, eyes straining with concentration in order to finish up and get out and play.

Suddenly the screen door leading from Peggy's bedroom to the back porch slammed shut with a crashing sound. Eight decibels of brisance spewed into the house. Nobody was supposed to be there but his own self. The Kid jumped, his skin crawling with goosebumps. Somebody had finally come to get him. He knew it. With absolute certainly.

All the lies he'd told. All the sins he committed. All the times he'd skipped Sunday School and church. A monster moulded in the image of all the Kid's wet beds and lies and thefts and bad thoughts and unworthy deeds.

It was going to be so bad he'd faint when he saw it. The hair on his arms and neck stood on end. His skin pricked. He was that far from the most horrible death there had ever been and he knew it. There was nothing he could do to prevent it. All he had was his crutches. And a monster that big and bad it wouldn't even feel it if the Kid whacked him with a crutch.

He waited. He quaked.

"Hello." He had to do something, so he softly called out a greeting.

"Hello." Again. "Is there anybody there?"

No answer.

He sat there cringing from the thousands of worms that were crawling all over him.

Listening. Listening.

Still not a peep.

He quietly reached over to retrieve his crutches which were leaning against the wall at the corner of his desk.

His entire body trembling, he stood up and quietly slipped his arms into the crutches.

And bravely but very, very quietly he tiptoed into the kitchen, as quiet as any herd of buffalo, so that he could see what — or who — had slammed that door.

Not wanting to. Not able not to.

161

Nothing.

He finally reached the door of Peggy's bedroom, stopped stock still, listened very carefully for a couple of minutes and only then stuck his head through the door, ready to withdraw it on the run at the first move of the monster to wrench his head from his body.

Where is it? Where is it? Which way can I run to get away? Will it kill me? Will it take me with it? Please, God, I'll be better about my prayers and I'll never miss church again and I'll pray five times a day, God, and give You all the credit for anything good that I ever do in my whole entire life.

What is there? He had to see. Can I stand to look at it?

He opened his eyes. And saw that the screen door was closed.

And saw nothing. And heard nothing.

No droppings. No spoor. No heaving breathing. Nowhere could the Kid find the thing God had sent down to scare him to death and eat him up.

It must be somewhere else! It's gotta be somewhere else.

He went through the house, knowing someone was there. Filled with trepidation.

The front bedroom was clear. Grandmother's bedroom. Not a peep.

The little room off her bedroom. Even in the repository of all the junk in the house, the ideal place for a marauding monster to hide, there was nothing. Nada.

Then he got real scared. Terror kicked the Kid into high gear.

What's worse than the ugliest monster that's bent on torturing, then eating mean-assed polio kids in Rorie Addition, west Paris, Tennessee?

The answer was easy. INVISIBLE MONSTERS! That are too ugly to be seen but who have the same strength and moral turpitude.

Jesus H. Christ on a crutch! They're everywhere! I just can't see them. Oh God, Oh God. Ohgodohgodohgodohgod. I'm dead.

He got out of that house as fast as his crutches could carry him. Two-pointing all the way. He set a modern day escape speed record getting to the front porch. Away from the whatever it was that he couldn't see but which he was certain was his enemy.

And still no sign.

He looked up and down the road hopefully searching for grandmother. By now he would eagerly have faced the wrath of grandmother for not having finished his homework then to take one step back into that house.

Exhausted, he sat heavily in a chair on the porch and forced himself to breathe. Ten minutes later he saw grandmother coming down the road.

By then he figured he felt much safer from the monster, thank you, than grandmother's wrath and decided he ought to go back into the study mode before she got to the house and started fussing at him. He grabbed his crutches and quickly four-pointed himself to the desk.

Every night, it seemed, grandmother and Ronald would play card games. Sometimes the rest of us would join in the card games or in a game of dominoes, but mostly it was he and she. You could see her face soften up when Ronald was around. Which is one more strange thing about why she allowed Uncle Ralph and Aunt Pearl to take him to raise.

Just as strange, perhaps, is why grandmother, who never really liked any of the Moody kids except Ronald, took them in for so long? She insisted all you had to do to get by in this world was to be honest and God-fearing and work hard. "You can't be afraid of hard work. That's the problem with this world today. Too many folks are skeered of hard work. Won't touch it. That's why they wind up on the welfare rolls. Not cause they can't. Cause they won't."

This said while grandmother was cashing monthly welfare checks on the Kid and his three siblings. She got checks to help out — twenty or thirty dollars a month — a head. Maybe that's why. (But whether she got that from the git-go I don't know.)

Granddaddy worked as long as he could and probably earned a bit more than bare subsistence. Later grandmother would draw social security. I suppose the minimum amount.

I don't know whether mom's siblings threw money into the kitty. I do know they and other members of the family periodically brought boxes of clothes for those poor little orphan kids Miz Sutton was taking care of.

Grandmother and others managed to get their hands on the insurance money mom's death had left for her four kids in trust. Except there was nobody to trust and nobody except Peggy and Ronald saw any of it.

The Henry County Clerk or the Henry County Probate Court or *somebody* in the Henry County Courthouse was supposed to have kept an eye on that money and hold it in trust for each of the kids until age twenty-one. Was that money at least partial motivation for grandmother letting the kids live with her and granddaddy?

The Polio Punk

Having polio wasn't nearly as much fun as the Kid wished it was. Oh, the attention he got, especially from adults, was wonderful and made him feel special. But mostly it sucked. Big time. The shoes, the plow shoes. The corset with its steel staves. And the crutches. How the hell could you live like a human being and be encumbered by those pieces of aluminum and wood stuck on your arms?

Walk down the street swinging hands with your favorite nine year old babe. Yeah, right. Squeezing her fingers between your hand and the handlebar of your right hand crutch. Until she screams in pain. And jerks away. And runs away. And never offers to do the sweet thang again. And tells all the other potential little sweeties about it so they, too, run away before you get a chance to court them.

To hell with 'em. He'd go back to the grownup women; they were prettier anyhow. And hugged better. And smelled better. And were a helluva lot sexier. The fact that there weren't that many nine year old babes in the neighborhood was probably a factor in this change of plan.

And what about those damn rules the grownups were always coming up with to "protect you from yourself." And chase away whatever chance the Kid had of making friends. "Don't run with those crutches, Kid. You'll ruin your legs and break the crutches." So what happens when the Kid walks? First thing is all the other kids start chasing after each other and before he can reach the end of the driveway with his fucking four-point gait they're all the way up to the top of the hill. Once in awhile one of the kids would stay behind for a minute in sympathy. "I'll walk with you, Kid." Yeah, long enough to figure out how damned boring it was. "I'll go on and wait for you in the field up there. Okay?" As if the Kid really had input.

"You gotta come in and take your nap, Kid; you can come out and play again in two hours." Two hours later there wasn't anybody to play with, not even if they were playing while sitting on their asses on the Kid's front porch.

The Kid's own kind of fun ranged from thumb-twiddling to thumb-sucking to (gently) patting the toes of one foot against the ground to a tune that welled from the inner recesses of his soul. Or the radio. The Kid did love music.

And then onto the exercises.

If he could have articulated the reason for his rage way back when, the Kid would have talked about feeling excluded from almost everything in life. He couldn't run and play. That's not saying the Kid never did. Oh, he was constantly on the lookout for chances and every chance he got he boogied to a fun place.

Later, when he got up enough nerve, he'd even play baseball with neighborhood kids. Drop one crutch. Lean on the other crutch. Swing the bat with both hands and when he made a hit, scoop down and pick up the crutch from the ground and lope to first base, swinging both legs in sweeping arcs as he rushed toward safety.

The Kid led, at least, two lives. Trying to stay reasonably within the rules when he was within sight of grandmother's prying eyes and trying to pack as much fun as he possibly could into the moments when he was not. Running and jumping and "acting a fool" as long as he thought he was safe from arrest. The truth was the Kid wasn't nearly as out of hand as grandmother imagined that he was. He mostly stayed close to home and studied and crammed his mind chock full of adventure. Most of the adventure of his life was confined to the thick, bony walls of his skull:

The Kid Flies to Mars: The trip took at least an hour by the time he got into his spacesuit, climbed into his rocket, checked everything out real carefully and hit the launch button. But what marvels he did behold along the way. Sometimes alien spaceships would dock with his rocket and he'd invite them in for a cold drink and a game of cards, and, of course, serious discussions about the state of the universe. Despite some close calls from meteors and unfriendly aliens the Kid always made it safely home, usually just in time to hear grandmother yell something about "paying attention." *What's wrong with her? I've just come back from Mars in a spaceship I personally designed and built. I've got a bucketful of samples from there that could change the way we think about the human race forever and she thinks I need to pay attention?*

Years later the Kid wondered how Peggy, Jacky and Ronald looked at his invading the space they had carved for themselves with grandmother and granddaddy. It hadn't occurred to him then that they might regard him as an intruder. And rightfully so. Everything was stretched even more tightly as a result of his being there. Space and money and love and grandparental temperament. And did he truly help to hasten granddaddy's death, as grandmother often insisted?

Although mostly it had just fucked up whatever shot the Kid had at a normal life, there were some polio plusses, too. He began reading, a lot. And when class-room work was thrown at him he took to it, really liked it. Probably because it warded off the deadly amalgam of boredom and loneliness that would sometimes pervade his being when he was idle, when he allowed himself to think about the reality of how rough his life had become.

Until he'd contracted polio, the Kid's world was a physical one. Polio forced the Kid's attentions to the sedentary joys because it was either have a good time while he sat on his ass or be miserable while he sat on his ass; the only thing about which there could be no doubt was that he would be sitting on his ass.

Besides, if he played his cards right schoolwork could even give the Kid bragging rights.

Memphis Magic

Aside from the megadoses of self-pity, the trips to Memphis generated a practical problem for those who would take credit for being good and kind to the Kid. How to get from point A, Henry County, to point B, the Shelby County outpatient polio clinic, when your family is fiscally flatter than a fritter?

The Kid's very existence depended on the piety of others. Nothing was "deserved". The Tennessee Department of Welfare threw in a few bucks a month to help them out. Somebody else paid for the time he had spent and the treatment he had been given at Isolation Hospital in Memphis, right after the bug hit him. The Kiwanians paid for the rehabilitation at Crippled Children's Hospital. Somebody, not family, paid for his corsets, shoes and crutches.

The little fucker had become a beggar, a seeker of life-sustaining handouts, and, instead of working his way out of it, had, by the age of ten, become deeply entrenched in walking the walk and talking the talk.

Piety. Charity with a twist.

As long as the Kid lived with Uncle Sam, money for the trips to Memphis didn't seem to be a major problem. The answer may be that Uncle Sam was getting financial aid from the March of Dimes or some other charitable group even then. Makes sense, if he was as broke as he claimed to be.

Either Uncle Sam would drive the psychedelic Dodge or would help Aunt Margaret drive her and Uncle Telous' car. Once when Aunt Margaret was driving one of her tires blew out. Uncle Sam was sitting in the passenger seat. He quickly reached across and grabbed the steering wheel to avoid an intermediate stop at another hospital.

The problem there was that whoever drove the Kid to Memphis had to miss a day of work. Aunt Margaret worked at the Salant and Salant Shirt Factory and had to take a vacation or sick day. Uncle Sam had to miss a day of farming.

After Uncle Sam's, the Kid found adventure of yet another kind. His treks to the most populous and most fascinating city in the Volunteer State switched from the highways to the railways. Grandmother and granddaddy had never owned more than a two mule powered vehicle in their lives, except for maybe a farm tractor. When they wanted to go somewhere grandmother said, "We can either use 'shank's mare' [feet] or borrow a ride with somebody."

Uncle Sam could no longer be asked ethically to do it because the Kid had slipped out from under his roof under a dark cloud of something or the other that affected all that, either in grandmother's mind or in reality.

Faced with the terrifying possibility of taking care of a total invalid — never mind that there was no basis in fact — grandmother found the solution. Seemed like every other house in Rorie Addition housed a worker for the L&N Railroad. So why not hit some of those folks up for chaperone duties for the Kid. And then, when he had the experience, he could do it by his own self.

She must have been a prophet.

That's exactly the way it happened.

Amazing.

The first trip after the flight from Uncle Sam's was under the aegis of Miz Markham. Lona Bell Markham, brazen wife of John Markham, engineer extraordinaire for the L&N Railroad Company. Kinda short. Kinda frizzy hair. Eyes aglitter and atwinkle. A live wire. Grandmother wasn't sure but talk was that Miz Markham had herself a drink of whiskey or beer once in awhile. She'd heard stories because both of 'em had been married before and everybody knew what that meant. Maybe it wasn't fittin' that the Kid should go with her because of her obvious bent toward sin.

But she did offer.

It was settled. The Kid could go with Miz Markham but he wasn't to talk about it when he got back. Not about who he went with. That would be too embarrassing to the "family". Not unless he had to say in order not to lie outright. "Just be sure to let me know if she takes you into one of them beer gardens. I won't have none of that." Grandmother was expert in the sneaky-pete approach to confronting people. She said what she had to say behind the back of the person she wanted to say it to.

Let the visits begin.

Let the Kid's chaperone checkup visits to Memphis begin.

Oh, yes. There was something else that had to be done before the Kid could go anywhere.

Green is the color of go

Somebody had to pay.

Grandmother said she couldn't afford it.

So she found the Henry County March of Dimes.

Grandmother's house was less than a half a mile from the railroad tracks. The night before his first train ride ever he had taken his bath. All he had to do was his exercises, put on his shoes, corset and clothes, wash the sleep off of his face, eat the oatmeal and toast grandmother had waiting for him and wait for Miz Markham to drive up the hill.

A car stopped in the gravel in front of the house. As he reached the car his head jerked back. Grandmother was there behind him! *What's she doing here? Get outta here. Go away.*

"I know this is going to a lot of trouble, but I wancha to know I really appreciate it. Much obliged 'til you're better paid." Grandmother's oft-repeated expression of appreciation when she didn't intend to pay anything at all. Translated, it comes out. "Take my thanks, 'cause you aren't gettin my money."

Grandmother climbed out of the car and the Kid got inside. And away they went! The two adventurers. On a mission of excitement through the corridors of the unknown to the chafing rooms of the polio clinic.

A mile away Miz Markham turned the car off Depot Street to park on the north side of the depot. Miz Markham bought the ticket. They only needed one for the Kid because Miz Markham's married to Mr. Markham and travels for free.

"We're early, Kid. Wanna go outside and sit on a bench out there where we can see the train when it pulls in?"

Lights are widely spaced along the skirt of the train station, casting a look of unreality on everything. Sound amplified tenfold at four o'clock in the morning in a deserted city. It echoed with startling eeriness. The Kid felt like he was dreaming. That he was an observer and not a participant. It was too good, too beautiful, too exciting to be real.

Until he saw the bright eye of a headlight shining through the early morning dewmist ahead of the loud rumbling of steel wheels against steel rails and the creaking of swaying cars slowing down as the engineer pulled sharply on his steam whistle, shattering the early morning quiet.

That's when he abandoned his role of uninvolvement. He could barely control his excitement at the first sight of a train so close up.

He could see there were dim lights on in some of the coaches giving life to the passengers scattered helter-skelter among the seats inside.

In moments he would join them.

A passenger.

On a train.

Thank you, God, for being so good to me. Joy. Joy. Joy!

Shivers ran up and down his back.

The train comes to a halt. Passenger cars alongside the ticket office. There's no platform. Paris isn't big enough for that. The conductor jumps off the train as it stops, picks up the footstool and places it under the bottom step leading up into the passenger car and motions the Kid up. The first step is no problem. The second step is a big problem. The conductor puts his hands under the Kid's arms and hoists him onto the main platform.

"All 'board!"

174

He stoops and picks the boarding stool up and, after a final glance, hops onto the platform, picks up a lantern and signals to the engineer that all is well in the place of passengerdom.

The train ride is a marvel; from the sound clickety clack, clickety clack, to the roar of steel moving swiftly over steel, coupled with a jerky side-to-side rocking motion, mixed with an occasional up and down grind and shake.

The Kid is awestruck. He doesn't blink more than once every five minutes during the more than four hour ride. Afraid he'll miss something. First there's the darkness. Then the lights. Illuminating mysteries of city and farm life. Lights shining through occasional farmhouse windows. The Kid knows that means the farmers are getting up for the morning chores but when you're speeding through the night in a magic car there's no ordinary anything. Everything takes on an excitement no matter how mundane it might have been yesterday, how boring it will be tomorrow.

Watching a small yellow light through the closed window of a house a hundred yards away at four o'clock in the morning is not far removed from high spy adventure. The agent keeping track of his quarry. And quietly. And resolutely. With the quarry, whose high crimes and misadventures are so very close to public disclosure, whose lives are moments away from total pathetic chaos. Unaware. Unsuspecting. And absolutely helpless to save themselves.

While the Kid contemplates the fate of the hapless folk whose crimes he's uncovered, he eats his meatloaf sandwiches. Actually, he eats one and hides the other so that Miz Markham will have to buy him dinner and sup-per from a restaurant. Grandmother may think it's fool-ish to spend money for food when you can get honest, wholesome food at home; the Kid prefers restaurant food. Anytime. All the time. And sneakery is not an un-acceptable price to pay for it.

The world slowly comes to life as the sun rises. To his delight the Kid finds there are just as many mysteries to be solved in the daylight as at night. Especially in the early morning when the guilty aren't able to conceal their shame as effectively as when the sun has climbed higher into the sky. Footsteps shuffling on the platforms of all the stations along the way.

It's just like in the movies. Steam boiling around the legs of men and women who have been conscripted by the Secret Service to pretend they're just ordinary res-idents of ordinary towns in the sleepy little vistas of west Tennessee.

But they forgot the Milan Arsenal, didn't they? Forgot to disguise it. Too late. The Kid knows it's all about making weapons and beating the Commies and warding off the Yellow Peril.

And he can see, with his nose pressed tightly against the window, what they're trying to do. He knows they can never do it without his help. And he has re-solved, in the two-and-a-half hours since the train left the Paris Depot, to help them. He will maintain the watch. He will be the early warning system. He will be the one who will warn them of imminent danger when the *others* expose themselves, as they must in those moments before they commit their heinous acts of tyranny. He will save them all.

If they attack before he and Miz Markham get off the train in Memphis.

This was easily the most exciting trip the Kid had ever taken.

Miz Markham mostly slept her way to Memphis. And she should have. The better to prepare her nerves for the site of Union Station in Memphis.

He was staggered by Union Station. A hundred, a thousand, times bigger than Paris. Fifty times louder. A gazillion times more exciting. A huge ornate building filled with a ceiling higher than the tallest building in Paris and decorated with mind boggling gargoyles and stained glass and marble floors. A restaurant. Picture-taking booths. The outside front carved from granite. And the backside where the trains came and left. It looked to the Kid as though there were a hundred tracks.

"We only have half an hour before your appointment, Kid, we'd better get out of here and get ourselves a cab so you won't be late."

"Yes ma'am.

What's that? Holy cow! I've never seen anything like that before. What are those people doing? Is that woman giving that colored man money? What for? Wonder if somebody will give me some money? Look at all the people, will ya! Every-where!

Voices amplified by echoes bouncing back and forth. The Kid had never heard so many voices speaking at the same time. Were any of them directed at him? He couldn't tell. He didn't know.

The cab driver got out of his cab, walked around to the passenger side and opened the backdoor for first Miz Markham to get in and then the Kid.

177

They were there on time. In time for the Kid to wait and be x-rayed and showed off and graded and cast off til the next time.

Another cab to an address Miz Markham gave the driver. A drive to the suburbs. To a ranch style home where they were greeted by a lady with a wooden leg. She gave Miz Markham a hug like they were long lost best buddies. And Miz Markham, who wasn't one to display a whole lot of emotion to anybody as far as the Kid had seen, hugged her right back.

All of which was fine with the Kid because the one-legged woman hustled him off to a television set!

The Kid made an important discovery in his life that day, a discovery that was to change his life thenceforth. And that was that watching television is like riding a bicycle. Once you've learned how, you've got the skill for life.

Snacks to go with the tube? Joy, oh joy, oh joy! The Kid wanted to stay here. The Kid had found himself a place of permanent comfort.

The Kid was a little beggar. Oh, he didn't just up and ask for things. He was more laid back than that, what he would later learn was called passive-aggressive. He'd just turn those baleful blue eyes on something and hang in there until some wonderfully obliging adult would see him and feel sorry and buy it for him. But the first time he went to Memphis with Miz Markham he came up dry. Of worldly goods, that is.

The train ride back to Paris didn't diminish his day one whet. It had been of the very best of his life.

There were other train trips to Memphis and other chaperones, including Miz Scholes. Miz Scholes was the church lady on the street. Every time the doors to West Paris Baptist Church opened Miz Scholes was there.

Before their last trip together, a time after the Kid started attending school, Miz Scholes invited the Kid to spend the night before at her house, for convenience's sake, so that they could just get up in the morning and leave and not have to worry about her picking him up in a cab.

To the train station. Boarded the train. Got to the Polio Packing Plant without a hitch. And then to the cafe across the street from Union Station for hamburgers and a strawberry malt. Miz Scholes wound up buying the Kid some cheap little treasure from the novelty gift shop next door to the scuzzy cafe.

He saw one of those little booths where you get pictures taken for a quarter. Go inside, sit on the little built-in stool-bench, close the curtains, insert a quarter and push go. Three shots. Three different poses.

But then what could he do with the pictures? Grandmother would be as mad as a wet hen if she ever found out he had wasted a quarter like that. Kept them with him as long as he could then threw them away.

The Kid learned the lure of coin returns. One day he pushed the coin return lever in the photo booth and got a quarter back. He started pushing every coin return he came across and during one trip collected nearly a dollar and a half. Which he promptly spent at the gift shop for neat stuff.

The threat of grandmother's verbal violence wasn't enough to deter the Kid from tasting and touching and generally experiencing every single delight he could find in his life.

Back to School

Fourth grade. The Kid was a part of the crowd that day. His first day in a real classroom since the first semester of the second grade. The fall term at Robert E. Lee Elementary School in Paris was more than a month old when the Kid was finally allowed to break away from his home studies and venture out into the flesh-and-blood-and-brick-and-mortar world of academia.

Arrangements had been made. He had to take a taxicab to and from class because he couldn't get in and out of a bus. He would come in late his first day so he wouldn't have to deal with the traffic in the halls and stairs. The other kids in school had to be cautioned not to fuck with him because he was "crippled" and crippled kids couldn't play like ordinary kids scuffle or run. Somebody figured it would be best if he didn't get there with the rest of the kids on the first day back so he didn't.

Miss Charlie, the principal, led him inside the classroom where he saw a bunch of strangers, all of whom were looking at him funny because he's a freak and laughing inside at him because he's a freak and hating him because he's crippled and because they'll have to play with him anyway because the teachers are gonna make 'em. The strangeness, the fear, the hostility hit him with the force of a blast furnace.

"Kid, this is your teacher Miz Craven."

He couldn't get himself settled. Not in geography class. And not in math class which followed. The only comforting sight he saw that first day back, besides the cab which came to take him away from all the fun and games, was Jacky marching up and down the hall with his sixth grade class. There was nothing like a big brother to protect you from that whole universe of estrangement. Jacky never physically came to the Kid's help, but his presence was comforting. If anyone did fuck with him he could run to big brother. For emergency use only, of course.

He'd never remembered this many kids in one place before. The Kid thought he'd died and awakened in a paradise. No, not a paradise yet, but a potential paradise.

The Kid rode in American cabs. Over the next couple of years the Kid would come to know all the American cabdrivers. They became a very comfortable part of his intimate environment. His family. It was like your big brother or sister or your dad or mom driving up to your doorstep every morning and afternoon. If someone else wasn't there to help the Kid the driver would jump out of the cab, come around and open the front passenger door with a flourish, like a doorman at a big hotel giving special service to a special guest. The Kid revelled in it.

As the days and weeks passed the Kid got back into the groove. Real school was not as hard as he'd been afraid it would be that first morning. The Kid was one of the three or four top grade getters by the end of the year. He also was finding it easier to climb the stairs, and even better, going down the stairs to recess and lunch and the waiting taxicab.

Once the strangeness had subsided, the Kid began to have the time of his life. He could walk with his hands and arms all the way across the monkey bars, much to his surprise.

Fourth grade was the last grade where there was only one teacher. Beginning with fifth grade, students had four. The students stayed in the same classroom all

181

day; it was the teachers who had to pack up their books and papers and traipse off to the next group of victims.

In fifth grade he was in Miss Mavin Miller's room. The Kid was drawn toward her. She had a kind of quiet magnetism, as if you knew she could lead you to some place you wanted to go. After lunch each afternoon she read to the class during the half hour of officially imposed quiet time.

"Heidi" is the ultimate punishment for a naive kid of what? Ten? Written by some sadist whose message is that no matter how brightly the diamond shines, when the glow is gone there's nothing left but a piece of rancid shit. First we're told about this wonderful little girl who goes to live with this wonderful little grandfather on the mountainside with his goats and Peter the goatherd. Peter and the goats are also wonderful. The cheese is wonderful. The stories are wonderful. The relationships are wonderful. There is no need for Trojans on grandfather's mountain because all is well.

Or would have been if the goddamn relatives hadn't jumped in to interfere. Just couldn't stand perfection. Had to jump into the middle of paradise and fuck it up. For the hell of it. No doubt that under that placid facade of magistral serenity lay a demon who had escaped from the depths of the devil's own hell and came to scare the shit out of little kids who wound up in Miss Miller's fifth grade rest period.

Now, if you wanted to look at the essence of evil on two feet, all you had to do was look at Miss Carter. She was by far the scariest teacher in Lee School and made no bones about what she'd do to you if you didn't follow all those rules she laid out for you at the beginning of the school year.

No subtlety. Like the time she caught the Kid staring into space during her fifth grade class one sunny spring afternoon, soaring over Paris with the buzzards and crows when she thought he should be paying attention to the textbook laying on the desk in front of him. Suddenly he felt this sharp, burning pain on his right hand.

Whap.

Whap.

The bitch had hit him! Hit him. Sneaked into his daydream. And hit him. The Kid had never been hit ever in school before. Never a switching, not even a spanking! Although he had gotten real close at Van Dyke one time in second grade. But there was no blemish on his record.

Until now.

Whap.

That ruler stung worse than a hornet.

The embarrassment of being hit by a ruler in front of people he was trying to impress as the perfect student and person was unendurable. Wishing, however, rarely seems to result in effective self-emulation.

"Pay attention, Kid. And the rest of you. You think these rules are for my benefit? If you're ever going to make anything of yourselves you're going to have to pay attention and not just in my class, but in every class you're ever going to take for the rest of your lives. You're either going to pay attention or be left behind under the wagon. If you think that's mean, so be it. I'm telling you for your own good."

The Kid sat up and paid attention.

For the next two years.

In Miss Carter's class.

Miss Carter and the Kid never met outside the classroom, except in passing on the streets and shops of Paris, once he'd left her homeroom. It took several dung beetle lifetimes for him to figure out that she was the antithesis of the ogress he had known her to be way back then, that she and Mrs. Ridgeway were the best teachers he had had the good luck to have.

The Kid reached his moral nadir in fifth grade. He was the first school safety patrol officer who operated on legs and crutches in Paris, Tennessee. First thing out of the cab he'd strap on his little white bandolier with the badge on it, toss his books onto the grass by the sidewalk leading to the front entrance, and go to work.

Work was stopping cars carrying students at the designated spot for disgorging. He worked with a will. Fearlessly, he'd stand in front of the oncoming automobiles, motioning them forward, then, when they got to exactly where he wanted them he'd throw up his arm, palm vertical. "Stop!"

He surely did enjoy his work. Being a school safety patrol officer was one of the first times after the attack of the evil viri that the Kid felt normal. Nobody telling him you can't do this or you can't do that. No adults getting in his way. He was a person not just a concession when he was standing there.

For most of his life thereafter whenever the Kid wanted to demonstrate his manliness he'd step into a street in front of traffic to show off how he could stop traffic at will. And, miraculously perhaps, never got hit.

The Kid took his safety belt home at night so that he wouldn't have to go inside the building before he took up his duty post in the morning. He'd just exit the cab and be ready to rock and roll.

One day the Kid stole a lieutenant badge from one of the safety patrol belts. He himself was a mere patrolman but he lusted mightily after that lieutenant badge. Patrolmen badges were plain aluminum but the lieutenant badge sported a bright blue field around the lettering which said "School Safety Patrol" with the rank stamped across the lower portion.

The Kid saw that lieutenant badge every day when he took his belt into Miss Charlie's office every morning to store it for the day. The more he saw it the more he wanted it. He really wanted it. One day he looked furtively around him, grabbed the belt, unpinned the badge with the magnetic field of blue and put it into his pants pocket.

He stole a school safety patrol lieutenant badge!

What a treasure!

Except after he had it in his pocket he didn't want it anymore. He couldn't wear it, somebody would see and know what he'd done. Grandmother would ask so many questions he'd be caught and tried and sentenced to a lifetime of embarrassment. He couldn't take it back because it never crossed his mind. So he gave it away. Just handed it over to Gayton Chilcutt, figuring Gayton would admire his chutzpah and add the badge to his collection of strangeness. Over a period of a year or so the Kid felt like he'd gotten close enough to Gayton to call him a buddy.

But Gayton told!

Gayton told!

Gayton told Miss Charlie!

Next morning Miss Charlie called the Kid into her office. Miss Charlie, sitting at her desk, looked up from what she was reading, opened the middle drawer of her desk, took something out and held it up for the Kid to see.

He near 'bout shat.

A school safety patrol lieutenant badge.

"What do you know about this, Kid?" Miss Charlie asked in a neutral voice, neither accusing nor praising.

"Nothing, Miss Charlie."

"I'll ask you once more. Did you take this from my office without permission? I might as well tell you that Gayton Chilcutt has already told me you gave it to him, so I suggest you make it easy on yourself. And, for your information, he didn't tattle. He was showing this around on the bus yesterday afternoon and another student told me about it. I talked to him. He told me about you. And you're here. Now, again, where did this come from, Kid?"

"From your office, Miss Charlie."

"Did you take it?"

"Yes ma'am."

"Why?"

"I don't know."

"You don't know why you stole from my office? Don't you know how serious that is, Kid? You could be expelled from school. As hard as you've worked to get back into school you wouldn't want that, now would you?"

"No ma'am."

"Can't you give me any reason for doing this?"

"No ma'am."

"This is very serious, Kid, but just this once I'm going to overlook it. By that I mean I won't call your grandmother in for a conference and I won't expel you from school. I won't even suspend you from the safety patrol for I know how much you like your work in it."

"But I'll be keeping my eye on you, Kid. What you've done is violated my trust in you, so now I must be watchful, careful to insure that you don't repeat something like this in the future."

"If you keep your nose clean by the end of the year I'll wipe your slate clean. If, however, you violate my trust again before the end of this year, I won't hesitate to use this badge as additional evidence against whatever you might get into your mind to do."

"Do you understand me?"

"Yes ma'am."

"Okay then, go back to class."

Miss Charlie didn't have to tell anyone what had happened. By the time the Kid returned to Miss Miller's classroom he could tell they all knew what he had done. They knew and he wanted to disappear through a crack in the ground. Where was a good earthquake when you need one?

Nobody ever teased him about it, but he could tell by the surreptitious glances when they thought he wasn't looking and by the giggles that he could hear behind his back and by the embarrassment that inflamed his soul.

And the truth of it all was that he had no idea why he'd stolen the damned badge!

The Kid was sure he was either going to die of humiliation or get caught by grandmother and skinned alive.

Weeks passed.

The trepidation that spilled over from his being into oatmeal slowly began to recede. First he noticed it wasn't making his oatmeal funny tasting anymore. Then he noticed he could relax for a few seconds once in awhile around grandmother. And then it slowly went away to its hiding place to wait for his next similarly senseless and inexplicable act of stupidity.

Some of the kids at school joined the 4-H Club. The Kid thought that would be cool. Those who lived on farms had cows and pigs and crops for projects for city slickers like the Kid. Grandmother said, "No, Kid, we can't afford it'"

The Kid didn't join 4-H.

There was a music room where the students sang. The Kid loved singing and when they offered lessons on musical instruments he lit up like a Christmas tree. He could see himself in a band uniform, marching down the streets of Paris on Mule Day, so proud and good and handsome. He forgot the crutches for a moment, but the return of his memory didn't deter him from bugging grandmother.

He had to buy a recorder, one of those plastic flute-like whistles for beginners, before he could take lessons. It's nominal, the teacher had said, but you must pay. From experience the Kid knew that asking grandmother to spend anything on anything was almost one hundred percent a guaranteed failure. Peggy was just about the only one who could prise money out of her. And Ronald, of course. Nevertheless the Kid finally found the courage to ask grandmother if he could please take music lessons at school.

"What's it cost?"

"Just for a recorder."

"How much?"

"Five dollars."

"I'm sorry, I'm truly sorry. But I can't grab money outta thin air and I shore can't find it nowhere else."

While the Kid was in fifth grade grandmother started letting the Kid travel on the train to Memphis for his checkups by himself. She figured he was old enough to take a cab to the Paris depot, get on the train, get off the train in Memphis, catch a taxi, go to the clinic, get out of the taxi, walk into the clinic, do checkup stuff, get a cab to the train station, wait for the train, board the train in Memphis, ride the train to Paris, get a taxi from the depot in Paris to grandmother's house.

And she was right.

Essentially.

He'd walk to the clinic in Memphis to save money, crutches and all. Didn't matter how tired he got. Didn't matter how scary the neighborhood he had to walk through was. Every time he walked he could save cab fare to spend on neat stuff like hamburgers and milkshakes and stuff from the gift shop. One time he bought a little souvenir scabbard knife. When he got home he hid it because he knew grandmother would raise hell and accuse him of stealing it. And when she found it in his closet under a pile of old clothes she proved him right. "Kid, whur'd you git this here knife?"

The Kid felt like somebody had hit him in the head with a two-by-four. Busted. *Why'd I ever buy that thing and bring it home. Now look at the mess I'm in. What can I say to make her go away? What am I gonna do? I can't tell her I walked from the train station to the clinic. She won't believe that anyways and even if she did she'd take my cab money away the next time and make me walk without a cent to spend on stuff. If I lie she'll find out. If I tell the truth she'll think it's a lie. Why'd I do it? Why'd I do it? What can I do?*

Paralyzed with panic. Of once again being stripped naked of everything but a big-ass neon sign on his forehead proclaiming his master sinner's deeds to the world, with copies special delivered to everyone he least wanted to know of his criminal personality. Of being discovered. He wanted to run away forever and ever to someplace where they'd never heard of him and his outlaw ways. "I found it at the train station in Memphis the last time I went for a checkup."

"Look at them eyes. You're lying to me agin, ain't choo, Kid. You know you didn't find this. You either stole it or somebody give it to you. Either way you shouldn't have it. Kid. Sometimes I don't thank ye'd know the truth if it hit ye in the head. Ye got too much yer daddy in ye to eebn know what the truth is, much less to tell it."

The confrontation with grandmother left the Kid as weak as a kitten, as it always did, as if he'd just gone through a hard day of basic training at Parris Island.

The fact of the Kid was, he wasn't a saint. What it was that saved him from himself was a lack of opportunity. The Kid would have made a king-sized thief if he had had the courage to back up his obsessive desire to steal. It made perfect sense to him that if you didn't have the money to buy the stuff then stealing was an acceptable alternative. If you could do it so you wouldn't get caught. And it seemed like he coveted near about everything he saw. Wishing and stealing and lusting and coveting were all part of the mulligan stew that teased the boy's hunger. Most every day of his life he would spend wishing for things and people he'd never have.

The Kid used to love sitting on those ornate wooden benches in the train station listening to the echoes of voices and footsteps bouncing off the cathedral ceiling and the high walls.

Later when he heard a recording of Paul Horn playing flute solo in the Taj Mahal, its notes reverberating for long seconds in soothing waves of diminishing sound before the next was struck softly, he was transported back in time in mind to Memphis Union Station and the sounds of clicking heels of shoes seeming to never end, for as one began to fade into far reaches of space and time another came in to fill the breach.

All this to a background of hushed human voices speaking in tongues, as though the train station was the modern musical equivalent to the Tower of Babel which Jesus freaks say the ancients built to reach heaven. Pissing off God with their overblown egotistical view of themselves, they wound up not being able to communicate with each other because God gave to them hundreds of different languages, effectively halting construction of the tower.

Except, inside the Union Station terminal the voices were melodious and soothing.

The Kid looked forward to his solitary trips to the clinic in Memphis.

One day as he was sitting in a hospital gown with his legs dangling from an examination table anticipating returning to the excitement of the train station, Doctor Ingram put his hands on the Kid's shoulders to check the progress of his scoliosis.

"We've found something that might help straighten up that back of yours, Kid. It's called a Milwaukee brace. It's got a leather girdle that is strapped around your hips with three steel staves, one in the front and two in the back, that hold leather pads that push up against your ribs to straighten your spine."

"The nurse tells me you've been traveling by yourself when you come for checkups. Is that true?"

"Yes sir."

"How do you get here?"

"On a train."

"Does that pose any problems for you?"

"No sir."

"How long have you been coming all alone?"

"Since fifth grade."

"We're going to measure you for a brace today and when it's ready you're going to have to come down and wear it home, but I don't think it's a good idea for you to come by yourself when you come down for the brace. You won't be able to move like you can with just the corset and crutches. It's going to be difficult for you to get around for awhile, until you get used to it."

"Do you think you could get someone to drive you down here then?"

"I think so."

"Tell you what, Kid. I'll call and make sure."

"Now off you go to the shop across the alley where you've been going to get your special shoes. The nurse will call over so they'll know why you're there. They'll fix you up."

"There's a good chance, Kid, that you'll be able to walk again without crutches. Wouldn't that be great?"

"Yessir."

"We'll all keep our fingers crossed. You're a pretty special little man around here."

The Kid didn't get back to the train station until late afternoon that day. The fitting had taken hours of measuring and pushing and pulling and twisting and torture. He took a cab because he was tired, but mostly because he was afraid he might miss his train if he walked to save the cab fare.

And back home. Home now consisted of grand-mother, Jacky and the Kid.

Ronald had gone to live with Uncle Ralph and Aunt Pearl. They'd met him down at Aunt Louise and Uncle Nolan's where he was spending a week away from grandmother once upon a time and took an instant liking to him. Not long afterwards, they drove to grand-mother's house and asked her if they might have the boy visit them for a few days of fresh air and farm atmos-phere. What could be healthier than that? Besides, they didn't have any children and they'd mightily enjoy hav-ing the tyke around for company.

Grandmother reluctantly assented.

And the hook was baited.

Two weeks later, they brought Ronald back and offered to give grandmother a helping hand by taking him off her hands permanently. They'd give him the kind of attention a child his age needed and would lighten her load, and, besides, they'd come to love the little guy during the two weeks he'd been at their house.

Ronald had a new home.

Until her dying day grandmother charged Aunt Pearl with poisoning Ronald against her during his first visit with them.

Aunt Pearl was Uncle Nolan's aunt. By marriage. I think. Grandmother said she had "reputation" because she'd been married more than once and "you know what that makes her." Uncle Ralph was a happy man with an insatiable sense of curiosity. White hair from the first time the Kid ever saw him. Twinkling eyes. Vigorous. Full of life. Always loud, always laughing. Always a joy to be around.

Years later Ronald told the Kid the reason Uncle Ralph had quit his job in Toledo, came down to Henry County and bought the farm was because someone, somewhere, had persuaded him there was money to be made. Profit. What a disappointment it must have been for Uncle Ralph to suffer year after year with little more than subsistence from the good earth of his beloved farm.

The irony is that Uncle Ralph and Aunt Pearl were themselves the treasures forever fondly remembered, especially by the children who knew them. There was something about them almost Pied Piperish. They drew kids like bears to honey. Perhaps because they had no children of their own, they reached out and touched children everywhere with moments of sheer delight. There was no pretense about either of them. They both talked naughtily sometimes to the delight of the young and to the chagrin of the not so young.

Both Jacky and the Kid would envy Ronald for the rest of their lives. He had escaped grandmother's perpetual fussing and fuming. They didn't. He got drawn into a life of fun. Of joy and laughter and intellectual stimulation. They didn't. He got to grow up with some semblance of normalcy. They didn't.

So Ronald had left by the time the Kid got his Milwaukee brace. And Peggy had gone off and eloped, marrying Joe Frankie Smith who worked at the ESSO gas station in east Paris. Peggy eloped in July of nineteen-fifty-four, the summer after her sophomore year at Grove High. And Jacky and the Kid knew it was because she wanted to get away from the harridan she called grandmother. And it was a lucky happenstance, they said, that she fell in love because she just might have taken off by herself to get out of there. Fifteen years old. And pretty as a picture.

This was the shape of the Kid's world before he went to town and strapped on his Milwaukee brace, preparing for his own version of the showdown at the not "ok corral". Early nineteen-fifty-five. The Kid went down to Memphis town where Doctor Ingram and company did a number on him.

Aunt Margaret and Uncle Sam had taken the day off work to drive him down in Aunt Margaret's Plymouth. The Kid had loved Aunt Margaret ever since he could remember, perhaps because she was the antithesis of grandmother. Aunt Margaret was gentle. Aunt Margaret was almost never seen to pick up a paintbrush dripping with venom and/or sarcasm. And she was the beauty of the Sutton siblings.

Down at the waiting room, fidgeting, first from boredom and then pain as it progressed from a thin line

196

of discomfort to full blown hacksaws being used to break somebody out from inside the Kid's ribcage.

Waiting.

The curtain parts. A pair of female hands reach in to pull the Kid into an examining room.

Waiting.

The dark frowning face of Doctor Ingram appears in the doorway. The frown changes into a kind of half-smile as his eyes fall on the Kid.

"Good morning, Kid. How're we doing today? Ready for the big day?"

"Yessir."

"Are you a little scared about wearing the brace?"

"Yessir."

"Well, don't be. It'll be fine and, in time, you'll be real glad you wore it. Okay?"

"Yessir."

The curtain is pushed aside by an aide to make way for a man carrying a strange contraption in his arms. Shiny metal and leather. Scary looking.

"Here it is, Kid. Your brand new Milwaukee Brace. Don't let the looks of it frighten you. I understand that it's actually quite comfortable. The only thing about it you might not like is that you won't be able to move around as much as you can now and you won't be able to bend your head down, so you'll have to be real careful when you walk. Keep watch ahead of you so you don't stumble over something in front of your feet."

"Understand?"

"Yessir"

"Okay, now take off your corset."

When the Kid was barebacked Doctor Ingram reached out and lifted him by the armpits from the examining table to the floor for his fitting.

The brace maker first strapped a heavy girdle around his hips. Covered with leather, the girdle seemed to be made of a metal frame fitted in with foam rubber padding covered by moleskin on the inside to lessen skin irritation over the months or years it would be worn. Three aluminum staves were anchored in its bowels. Two stuck up from the back on either side of the Kid's spine and one in the center of the front.

"There. That's not so bad, is it?" Doctor Ingram.

"Nossir."

"How does it feel? Is it too tight?" The brace maker.

"Nossir." The truth was the brace felt so strange the Kid didn't know whether to shit or fly. *I don't know whether it's too tight or not. I don't know how it's supposed to feel. I guess they know best, so I'll just go along with whatever they say unless it hurts me so bad I can't stand it. How's it supposed to feel?*

"Okay, if that's comfortable for you, let's put on the collar."

First a black headrest is attached. It will provide support for the Kid's head. It's attached to two staves which are attached to the girdle's rear staves by screws and wingnuts after Doctor Ingram decides how high the head should be raised to begin the spine-straightening process.

Then the chin rest, a small aluminum shelf covered by foam rubber covered by leather. Attached to the central front stave with yet more screws.

Finally Doctor Ingram steps back to look at his handiwork.

"I think that'll do it. It looks good on you. Kid. You're going to be the envy of all the kids in your neighborhood. It's not so bad, now, is it?"

"Nossir." The Kid's neck was stretched so far that he could hardly talk but he figured that's what they wanted. It didn't matter that there was discomfort, only that it was going to make him normal again. What the hell! It wasn't like they were going to give him a shot or anything like that.

Hadn't the doctor said the miracle Milwaukee Brace would straighten the Kid's back? It didn't matter if it pushed his head up til it hurt or if he couldn't look down or if it was uncomfortable as all getout. The Kid already saw himself set free of the restrictive bonds of polio. No more crutches. No more limping. No more slouching when I'm not wearing my corset. All I've gotta do is wear this thing until it straightens my back and I'll be like everybody else. Who cares how it feels now.

"Okay, Kid, you can get dressed now and I want you back here in a month so we can see how you're doing. Did you bring bigger clothes like I told you? That'll fit around the girdle and the staves."

"Alright, I've got to run now. I'll see you in a month." The doctor swirled and swept out of the examination room, leaving the Kid and Uncle Sam to ponder infinity since the Kid, for one, could no longer ponder his toes. They met Aunt Margaret in the waiting room.

Aunt Margaret and the Kid waited outside the clinic while Uncle Sam went to get the car, and away they went, stopping only for gas and for a wonderfully greasy hamburger.

Back to school the next day where Miss Charlie had assumed he'd have to give up his safety patrol duties. "No ma'am," he assured her. "I can still do it. I promise."

Reluctantly she allowed him to don his badge of traffic stopping authority and accompanied him to his post to see how well he could do it around his newfangled hardware.

He did it! He could still stop cars, the cars that didn't stop first to gawk at his get-up. And make the world of the area around the front entrance of Robert E. Lee School safe for little boys and girls of all ages up to and including the sixth grade. Safe from speeding automobiles and any other evil that might be lurking about.

He did it! Miss Charlie made her report to grandmother, who reluctantly gave her permission for him to resume his patrol role.

Adaptations quickly became a way of life for the Kid at school as well as at home. The first concession to which the Kid wouldn't give a second thought was that there would no bathing of the body inside the girdle around his hips. For a month. There would be no unbuckling of the girdle for any reason. Period. At school in Miss Carter's classroom, the Kid found he couldn't sit at a regular desk. The brace's staves fore and aft made him too big for the desk and even if he could have sat in one he couldn't see the top of the desk from eyes that were perched atop a head that was shoved skyward. Miss Carter was nothing if not inventive. She sent one of the students to the music room for a music stand, jacked it up to head level as the Kid sat in a real hard wooden chair, and, voila, there it was, a remedy.

Miss Carter also assigned different students to provide the Kid assistance through the day as he required it. To pick up papers, books and pens he dropped and to accompany him wherever he went in case he needed help.

Jacky was the designated helper at home. Mostly, the help the Kid needed was getting up when he fell and in the beginning he fell often because he couldn't see his feet. Once he adjusted to the different way of life, his clumsiness diminished considerably, e.g., he learned to memorize the path in front of him so that he could see it clearly in his mind's eye. He also learned to move with greater agility with the added handicap of the bulk and limitations imposed by the brace.

The Kid did not eschew all the new attention the monster brace brought his way. Far from it, he wallowed in it. If it had been sunshine he woulda had third degree burns over ninety percent of his body from preening in the spotlight. Everybody loved him and went out of their way to help him. And, most importantly, everybody went out of their way to say something to him every day. He couldn't have bought the kind of goodwill his Milwaukee brace brought him, but he would have if he could have.

However, while the Kid maintained what he thought was a demeanor of normalcy at school, the truth was it was not an easy adjustment. Not easy at all. Do you know how hard it is to write on a flimsy aluminum music stand? Or to move? Or go to the bathroom? Or to play safety patrol hero? Or eat without making a mess because he couldn't see the plate unless it was two or three feet in front of him and then the journey from plate to palate was perilous, interrupted often by spillage and fumble-fingered dumping?

Oh, he'd rather be in school than stay at home — that's for sure — but sometimes he thought life could have been a little easier had he not. Life was a whole lot less fun with his Milwaukee Brace putting the kibosh on just about anything the Kid wanted to do for fun. He spent an increasing amount of time sitting in one of the wooden rockers on the front porch.

Jacky, as always, was sympathetic and willing to help whenever he was around. Jacky had a big heart with a lot of love inside it but had as many emotional problems as it took to get him as fucked up as he would be most of his life. The Kid loved him, even when he was picking fights he knew he was going to lose because Jacky was built like a wrestler and the Kid was built like a string bean. Jacky, however, wasn't around anymore than he had to be on account of he couldn't stand grandmother's accusations and fussings and dissatisfactions with anything that remotely could be tied to the Moody clan.

The Kid went back to Memphis after a month. He thought he'd be back that night. He didn't return to grandmother's house for more than fifteen months.

"You can go home, Kid, and have some fun while you're waiting for your fusion."

The Kid felt like he'd been sucker punched in the belly. No way he wanted to go home. It wasn't a favor to send him back to that snakepit of anger and petulance and unhappiness.

"I haven't been feeling too good. Do you think I should stay until I feel better?"

"Let me have a look at you and we'll just see what the problem is."

Doctor Ingram looked and came up diagnosisless. "There is nothing I can find. Probably a case of homesickness. You're fit as a fiddle. A trip back to Paris is just what you need to get feeling bright and bushy-tailed. Don't you think?"

The pain from the punch spread.

The Kid felt trapped. His lungs felt like they were filled with cotton. Dread cast its net over his soul and caught him just as surely as if he'd been caught on the wrong side of a struggle to the death in the Coliseum of ancient Rome. Stupid. Stupid for not figuring out a way to stay in the hospital until....until he was grown or didn't have to go back to grandmother. He was desperate to turn the decision to send him home around. And completely helpless. *Can't they understand I don't want to go home? I hate home. I want to stay here.*

The old familiar sense of dislocation and isolation flooded the Kid, fogging his brain until he could hardly understand what was going on around him. *They can't, they just can't.*

The Kid had been admitted several weeks previously to Crippled Children's Hospital. He had taken to it like a duck to water. Just like he remembered from the first time, except it wasn't scary now. Miz Bean was still there taking care of the colored kids in the downstairs wards, but still coming up to visit him often. Miss Deming was still there, still working the midnight shift and still as sweet and kind as she could be - it seemed to him that every single one of those kazillion wrinkles on her face was a smile line. He was sure glad to be back. It was his most favorite place in the world. He had friends here. The nurses and the aides and the maids and everybody loved him; even the warden. And he loved them. And he didn't want to trade the cocoon of Crippled Children's Hospital for grandmother or for anything.

Unless, of course, grandmother had a sudden change of attitude so that she wouldn't hate Connie Moody and his kids so much. Unless, suddenly, she became a Miss Deming. That'd be cool. She wouldn't make you feel like she regretted every bite of food, every stitch of clothing and every other thing you had to be given. And it wasn't *only* because grandmother's was a bad home, but that it was easily eclipsed by the comforts and human warmth offered to children usually needy in both departments by hospital personnel.

Then there was the part about nobody being poor at the hospital. Everybody got sweets, got to see neat movies twice a week, television every day and cokes when your folks sent you nickels [thanks to Peggy and Joe Frankie.]

"Call his grandmother and tell her they can pick him up next Wednesday." Doctor Ingram told Miss Mason, the nurse. "His spinal fusion isn't scheduled until May, is it?"

"No doctor."

Miss Mason lived at the hospital. She had a little room off the rotunda just inside the entrance. Within two days the Kid had squeezed her out of her own room. Quarantined! Conjunctivitis! Pink Eye! *Praise Jesus. He listened to my prayer. Hot Dog!*

Soon as he got back to the ward the day of "the sentence", he started poking his fingers in his eyes. Under the eyelids. Til they were raw. Then he complained about his eyes hurting. Then they examined him and found conjunctivitis. The Kid had saved himself with a dose of the PINKEYE!

And nobody would ever know.

Peggy later told him the hospital had squealed on him, that they'd told them it was obvious that the Kid did not want to go home from the hospital. "They say the reason you didn't go home that time was because you didn't want to go home."

To which he proffered no reply. What could he say? Guilty as charged. And he knew whatever they did to him was less than he deserved.

And then he thought about the fun he was having.

His return to Crippled Children's had begun as a simple short stay to enable his handlers to check out the fit and efficacy of the Kid's Milwaukee Brace.

Get him in. Check him out. Send him home.

One two three.

Noper.

Check him out. Get this thing fitting properly. Ooops, let's have another look tomorrow; can he stay with us for a few days over at Crippled Children's? Fine. That will give us an opportunity to give more tests and see just how he is responding.

More tests.

Oh. Oh.

This brace thing isn't doing its duty. No way in hell it's going to straighten him up. Going to have to operate. Open up that boy's back and straighten out that scoliosis manually and brace it up with a stick of sheep bone. That's even better than shoving it up his ass, isn't it?

Having his own room was a trip for the Kid. Especially that part about special and individual attention. Hell, he coulda lived out his life in that neat little cubby hole. Not having to worry about going back home. Listening to Miss Mason's radio which she'd graciously left him while she went upstairs to the living quarters of aides and other employees who lived where they worked.

Among the aural acts at night was Oral Roberts, the Pentecostal. The Kid heard Brother Roberts pray to heal all them folk what was messed up. "Put your hands on the radio and believe. If you believe God will heal you!" The Kid put his hands on that little ivory-colored plastic radio every night. And believed. Real hard. That God was gonna heal him.

After a few days when it was obvious that it hadn't worked, Brother Roberts explained that sometimes, "if you don't believe sincerely with all your heart and soul God will not heal, but it's not God that has let you down my friends. No. It is you who have let God down."

Brother Roberts told the Kid [and hundreds of thousands of other listeners] that if the hands-on-the-radio didn't heal you what you probably need is a prayer cloth, a genuine prayer cloth for a donation of just a dollar. The Kid scraped together a dollar and sent it forthwith to Brother Roberts because he knew there was a way, someway, to get himself healed and back to normal and he was going to do everything he could to make that come true.

A few days later, while he was still in Miss Mason's room, the Kid got his prayer cloth from the reverend. A one-and-a-half inch square of felt. Felt! The same stuff they glue to the bottom of chess pieces.

This was it. Now or never. If he was good enough, God was gonna heal him now. He just knew it. He grabbed that little green square and squeezed it in his fist while he closed his eyes and prayed until his mind was drained. Until he couldn't think of another thing to add to the exhortations, the pleas to God to heal him and he'd be the best person there ever was that ever lived on planet earth. *If you will only see fit to heal me.*

Not long after that prayer, Doctor Ingram scheduled the Kid's spinal fusion for a day in May in nineteen-fifty-five at LeBonheur Hospital across town.

The days between were filled with pleasure for the Kid. He had finished the sixth grade under the watchful eye of Miss Graves. He won a book reading contest — thirty books in thirty days — and got a bible for his prize. He enjoyed his friends in the boys ward. He enjoyed being around all the women from aides to nurses to therapists to visitors. Yessir the little bugger could feel the sap rising even though, in truth, he had no idea what the hell it was.

Then.

There came the day when Leon piled the Kid onto a stretcher and pushed him out of the hospital to the station wagon for a journey to another hospital. "You'll be back here before you know it," he said through that warped grin of his.

He left Leon at the door of LeBonheur as a strange lady pushed him through the door to the place where Doctor Ingram had told him he was going to get a lot better. "You may even be able to walk without crutches!"

Eager but apprehensive.

Apprehensive but eager.

The lady left him on a bed in a room. There was no one else there. Which gave him a sense of isolation in contrast to how he felt cozy alone in Miss Mason's room. Miss Mason, with her stiffly starched white cotton uniform over the white stockings and under the white nurse's cap with the cute little pin that served as her bona fides.

At LeBonheur he felt alone and shivery.

"Hey Kid, how are you? My name is Mary and I'm gonna help you get ready for your operation tomorrow. I'm gonna shave your back, so they won't be getting any hairs into your incision. Want to roll over for me? That's right. Now this is not going to hurt a bit. I see you're all tensed up, but I promise you this is not going to hurt a bit. If you'll keep still. If you jump while I'm shaving you this razor just might nick you. So hold still."

Mary lathered up the soap in a shaving mug and spread the cool foam all over the Kid's back. Then shaved it. It felt good.

"So far, so good?"

"Yes ma'am."

She rinsed him off, dried his back, picked up the tray and left the room.

"Good luck tomorrow."

The Kid's bones felt like they were shivering. He'd brought his Bible with him. White leatherette with those soft thin pages that he loved to turn. He picked it up from the bedside table and turned the pages, reading here and there as he went, looking for something to take his mind off what he thought might not be such a wonderful adventure.

He knew the needles were coming. He knew they were going to hurt him again. He knew it and you could cut the dread that filled him with a dull sabre saw.

The Kid was scared and it was getting worse.

Afternoon. Four white coats came in, pushing a tray with the needle and a bunch of other apparati on it. All the Kid saw was the needle.

"Hi Kid. We are here to get you ready for your operation tomorrow. How you doing?"

"Okay, I guess." By now he was shivering from naked terror.

"This is not going to be real comfortable, I'm afraid, but we will be as gentle as we can be and get it over with as quickly as we can and still do a good job because we can't do it twice."

"What we are going to do is shoot some dye down the middle of your back so the surgeon will know where to line up your spine when he straightens it tomorrow morning. So this is very important. Can you be brave long enough for us to do it if we're as careful as we can be?"

"Okay." The Kid was shaking no less than if he'd been sitting naked on a frost-covered porch step in twenty-five degree weather.

"You have got to calm down a little bit now so we can do this without making it worse and without messing up," came the soft voice of the inquisitor.

"Try to relax. You can do it. Take a couple of deep breaths to get you started."

"Alright?"

"I'm really trying."

"I know. We all know how scary it is, but I promise you it won't be as bad as you think it will be. Here we go. Don't move. No matter what happens, Kid, don't move or we will have to start all over again."

They turned the Kid onto his stomach and wiped his back with gauze dipped in ether. The Kid gagged but soon forgot his nausea. It was buried by other, far menacing demons. He felt a sharp pain as the needle was inserted under the skin of the middle of his back. It hurt like the dickens, but he knew he could endure it.

"I know it hurts, Kid. I know it does. But it will be over in just a minute. Hang in there, we'll be done as quickly as we can."

Then they got serious. When they started pushing the bright blue dye from the syringe into his body he knew he had come face to face with the worst fear he had ever imagined. Nothing in his young life had prepared him for the onslaught of that awful pain.

Pain beyond words. Pain beyond imagination. Pain beyond belief. And with each newly discovered depth of unendurable horror, it got worse, so bad that his mind blanked out the pain to save his sanity. He felt no pain. Or at least no pain like he'd felt before. It was now pressure. What happens beyond pain.

It was if they were pushing a bulldozer through his backbone to the back of his head. He was sure he wouldn't, he couldn't, live through it.

"Good boy, Kid. You were brave. You did a good job. You should be proud of yourself."

"Get some rest now."

"Don't be scared when you go to the bathroom and see your urine is blue. It's from the dye we injected in there and it's perfectly normal."

They pushed their torture cart from the room and quietly closed the door. The Kid, exhausted from the ordeal of the past few minutes, fell asleep before the pain had gone away.

And woke up after dark.

The corridor lights were on, a sickly green from the combination institutional green walls and the fluorescent lights.

Absolute quiet.

The Kid woke up scared to death from the apprehension of the pain the morning would bring.

211

And alone. Not a soul he knew was anywhere near LeBonheur. His folks were in Paris and Henry County. His friends and the grownups he loved were at Crippled Children's Hospital.

The Kid was alone in these last hours before his operation. And that's exactly what it felt like. Nowhere to turn for solace. No one to chase away the ghosts of fear. No one.

And it was true. His pee was bright blue, the exact color of the blueing that Rena Mae used to whiten her clothes.

"Good morning!" The Kid jerked upon seeing the bright smile of a nurse bearing down on him from two o'clock. And managed a grin in return. Until he saw what it was she had on the tray she'd set on the bedside table top.

"Just a little shot to relax you before you go into the operating room. Won't hurt a bit, and it'll make you feel a whole lot more comfortable."

"Relax your arm now."

"All of this is for your own good. You may be in discomfort today and for a few days, but pretty soon you are going to be like new, almost like you never even had polio. Try to think about the improvement you're going to notice. You will be able to stand straighter. You may not even have to wear the corset anymore. And walk better. Wouldn't you like to be able to walk without your crutches? And just plain old feel better?"

"I will see you after you come back to the room this afternoon or tomorrow morning to check on how you're doing. Good luck today although from what the doctors have told me you don't need luck because it's for sure going to be alright."

The world started to relax around the Kid about then. His tight stomach loosened up. His worries about the operation and all the pain it was going to bring didn't evaporate but it did stop pounding him with its claw hammer.

It was a beautiful, sunshiny day.

In came the stretcher. Accompanied by a man and a woman, both dressed in green scrubs with white masks and skullcaps.

"Hey, Kid, you ready to get this thing on the road?"

"Yes ma'am, I reckon."

"Okay, let us help you up onto this stretcher and we will take a ride up to see the doctor."

Up the elevator through two sets of swinging doors into a room that would have scared him to death, making the spinal fusion totally unnecessary, if he hadn't been given that happy juice intramuscularly.

Shiny steel and aluminum everywhere. Bright lights. Must have been a dozen lights over the table they transferred him to; one at his shoulders and the other his feet. And in between.

And it seemed like a dozen people. Nobody talking to him. Everybody talking quietly to each other. Not about the operation, but about their kids and the weather and breakfast and the weekend.

The Kid watched and listened vicariously, as if he were monitoring somebody else.

The doctor came in. The Kid recognized who he was by his voice.

"Hey, Kid. Looks like we're all ready here. How about you? We're going to do a good job. Don't you worry. I'll be doing the operation so you're in good hands."

"First thing is the man here is going to insert a small needle in your arm so that we can get some sodium pentothal in you. He's called an anesthesiologist and he'll be taking care of you while you're asleep in here."

The needle slid in.

A pinprick of pain.

The Kid still didn't mind.

"Now what I want you to do for me is to count backwards. Can you count backwards from one hundred?"

"Yessir"

"Good. Start right now and take your time. Let's see how far back you can go."

"One hundred."

"Ninety-nine."

"Ninety-eight."

"Ninety-seven."

"Ninety-six."

"Ninety-five."

"Ninety-four."

The next thing the Kid knew he was retching in his bed back in his room. He would have been puking, except they hadn't let him eat anything. So now he was just practicing. In exaggerated fashion. His stomach heaving in and out in waves of nausea in what seemed like his passport to that heaven Oral Roberts was always preaching about.

Sick? The Kid was as sick as a horse.

His back felt like somebody was holding a red-hot branding iron to it. Dimly he saw Peggy and Joe Frankie sitting by the bed. Peggy leaned over. "Hi Kid. We're here. Joe Frankie is over there. And we brought you some comic books."

"Do you hear me?"

The Kid nodded.

With the nod came another assault of nausea. Someone brought some ginger ale from somewhere. He drank a couple of swallows.

And immediately puked it up.

"Don't talk," said Peggy. "You know we're here. If we're gone when you wake back up, we'll be back soon as we can. You know that, don't you?"

The Kid thought he nodded. But Peggy told him, later, he was too busy being sick to do much of anything.

A white uniform holding up two arms, one holding a syringe. "This will put you to sleep for awhile, Kid, and let you get some rest."

The Kid, who was scared shitless of hypodermic needles, hardly felt the prick of pain. When he awoke, the first thing he noticed was that Peggy wasn't there.

The second thing he noticed was the iron searing his back.

He screamed.

Begging for a shot.

Or anything else they had to push the pain away.

And so it went for a week. Wake up to the pain of his spine being removed from his body, take a few sips of ginger ale, scream for a shot, thence to sweet oblivion. He couldn't eat or read. He couldn't think over the din of his agony.

When Leon drove him back to Cripple Children's Hospital the pain was still searing. He expected they, too, would come running with a hypo when he couldn't stand it anymore.

Wrong!

They brought aspirin.

"I need a shot."

"You're not getting any more shots, Kid. You've got to get through this on your own. It's for your own good. Now take this aspirin and quit acting like a baby."

"It hurts really bad!"

"I know it hurts, but I also know it's not as bad as you think it is. Now take this and go to sleep. This'll all be over before you know it. They wouldn't have sent you back over here if you still needed the shots."

"Lie down now and try to rest. That's the best thing for you."

For two weeks the Kid was in almost constant pain and terror of the pain which sought to be soothed by those bullshit little pills that brought absolutely no relief. Ever. Every day he knew he couldn't get through another day. Or the next. Or the next.

Until one day it subsided; the dragon retreated into its cave far away in the mountains somewhere, leaving only hints of its presence.

The next fifteen months, almost all of which he would spend lying in a hospital bed, would also be perhaps the most joyful in the Kid's life. Hell, what was there not to like. Pretty women all over the place. Attention. Coca Cola on Sunday night (when he had a nickel). Movies twice a week. Visits from movie and tv stars: Superman; Sheena, Queen of the Jungle; Tim Holt, World's All-Around Cowboy.

Felt good! Didn't care if it was from the bed.

Oblivious to the world outside his cozy little private universe, the Kid purred with sensuous delight under the spotlight of ego gratification. What could be better than to be the poor little crippled boy confined to a hospital for all those months? "Poor little baby. I feel so sorry for him."

The little feller was not as poor as everybody thought he was. Hadn't he instigated the escape from the log house in Whitlock? Hadn't he sneaked around and peeked around and conspired and rebelled ever since? Mean fuckin' kid is what he was. On vacation for a minute from his reputation. Loving the attention and the limelight that he attracted.

It was the Kid who helped Richard and the other kid escape from the boy's ward. Richard, who had one of his legs tied up so he couldn't put any weight on it. TB of the bone, or something like that. And the other kid who'd been badly burned on every part of his body. Both wanted out. Both were tired of being cooped up in the hospital.

Doctors wouldn't release either one of them. So one night, after lights out, the Kid and Richard, whispering to avoid attracting the attention of the night aide, created an escape plan. The burned kid overheard them and threatened to tell if they didn't include him. Escape was never an option for the Kid because he couldn't get out of bed, but planning an escape, rebelling against authority in almost any form, was pure pleasure for him and the danger of discovery a savored stimulus.

It had to be in the early morning so they would have some daylight. Between the time Miss Deming brought them their toothbrushes and the time, twenty to thirty minutes later, that the morning maid came to work — no later than ten-of-seven — and started her rounds to pick up the toothbrushes and basins and cups and check to make sure every patient had indeed brushed.

The fire escape was on the other side of Richard's bed. A slide accessible by a high doorway that could be reached only by standing on the nearby windowsill or by climbing onto the lower part of the frame which was three feet or so off the floor or by reaching from a hospital bed.

"Now here's what you're going to have to do. Do you have any money?"

"Yes." The burned kid.

"A little." Richard.

"Well, you've got to have enough money for a cab or you'll never make it anywhere."

"I can take a bus because I live in town." Richard whispered.

"I'll take a cab." The burned kid.

"Miss Deming goes from here to the babies' ward. Richard, as soon as she leaves, you reach over and open the door. You'll have to take your crutches and your leg sling, though, so you can get on the street if you're going to take a bus. Anyway, both of you slide down the fire escape and take off. I'll get somebody here to close the door after you and you'll have half an hour or so to get away."

"Okay?"

"Okay!"

"Okay!"

"Tomorrow morning."

A whisper carries in the ghostly blue quiet of a hospital ward, though, and everyone in the ward was in the know as soon as there was a know, except for a few kids over in the far corner. Nobody slept a lot that night. Rasping wisps of conspiratorial delight floated back and forth. There wasn't anything more thrilling to those boys than the thought, the hope, the prayer that somebody could actually get away from there.

They waited.

And waited.

Until dawn began to creep through the ward's big windows, including the one in the fire escape door.

Until Miss Deming finally showed up to put them all to work on their teeth.

"Miss Deming! You know what Richard's gonna do?"

"Miss Deming I spilled my basin!"

Misdirection. And it worked.

219

The first boy's tattletale was quickly covered by another's quick thinking as a third shushed the would-be blabbermouth. "Shut up or you're going to get us all in trouble, including you."

As soon as Miss Deming left and made her right hand turn toward the babies' ward Richard made his move. He had already donned his leg sling and hooked his leg in it. He jumped up, hopped one-legged to the fire escape, pulled the door open, grabbed his crutches, stuck his legs out and started down the one-and-a-half story slide. Escape was being accomplished. The burn kid jumped on right behind him. In an eye blink both were gone. Another boy, who'd been assigned the task by the Kid, got out of bed and closed the fire escape door.

Perfect.

Nothing out of place.

Everything looked totally normal.

If you didn't count two empty beds.

Minutes passed.

Someone sighed.

The escape was a success. There is hope for the world. Indeed if there be escape from Crippled Children's Hospital, nothing is beyond the grasp of us mortals. Praise Jesus! Two-thirds of the patients in the boys ward were with the runaway pair every step of the way, running and hobbling and stumbling every inch of the way to the bus stop and taxicab.

Just as the morning maid walked in to start picking up the spit basins and water cups the kids heard a rapping sound on a window. They turned toward the fire

220

escape to see Richard's face pressing against the pane, knocking and frantically trying to get back in.

The maid heard it, too. She walked over, opened the door to the fire escape. "Whatchoo doin' out here, boy? Whatchoo thank y'all doin? Come on in outta dere." Richard didn't reply, didn't need to, the sheepish look on his face pretty much told the story. The morning maid was not a small person; she was not a short person; she was a big, strong person, who lifted Richard bodily into the room as if he were a lightweight jacket and carried him to his bed. She could have easily shotput him there, but chose restraint.

Richard had pulled himself back up the fire escape, no easy feat considering how slippery it was.

"You know y'all not s'pposed to be outta bed without yo crutches, boy. Where they at?"

"The bottom of the fire escape."

"Just havin' a little fun."

The maid scurried off in search of Miss Deming.

"I just couldn't do it." Richard quickly whispered. "I got to the corner of the building and just couldn't make myself go any further, so I came back. It was scary. I didn't think it would be, but it was really scary being out there all by myself. I did not want to get on no bus. And I was shivering from the cold. It wudn't all that much fun, to tell the truth. I ain't doin' that no more. I tell you!"

As she entered the ward another kid called out, "Miss Deming, the burn kid's gone, too!"

With one still missing, Miss Deming raced down the hall to awaken Miss Mason. By now the place was wide awake.

The police were called. "We've lost a patient. You can identify him from his burn scars and his pajamas."

Miss Mason strutted her stiffly-starched uniformed self around the ward, stopping at each occupied bed to ask "What do you know about this?"

The Kid said he'd heard something about it but didn't think it was serious.

"Why didn't you tell somebody, Kid? You are the oldest here. It is your responsibility to take care of the younger ones and to make sure they don't get themselves into trouble. Do you not know that Richard could have hurt himself seriously if he'd tried to walk on his other leg? Don't you know that the other boy needs treatment for his burns every day and that without that treatment he could get an infection or have some other serious problems? I count on you, Kid, to help us out with the others. I'm disappointed."

If you only knew I hatched up the plan, you'd really be disappointed. What have I done? Gotten myself into it again. What if she finds out? What'll they do? Send me home? Ooooooh!

The maid was dispatched to fetch Richard's crutches. She had to use the front entrance and walk all the way around to the back.

About the time the kids thought the burn kid had made it, he was ushered into the ward by Miss Mason. "Here's the other one. Now all you kids pay attention. This is serious. These boys could have been hurt or could have hurt themselves by running off alone like this. This is not a prison; it's a hospital. You are here for your own benefit. Why in the world would you want to escape? Aren't we good to you? Don't you like it here? You're

222

here to get better and when you get better you get to go home. But you cannot get any better by pulling crazy stunts like sliding down the fire escape at six o'clock in the morning."

Obviously exasperated, she walked out of the ward.

"What happened? How'd you get caught? We thought you were home free!"

"I got out to Lamar Avenue and even got a cab, but after we'd gone a few blocks the cabdriver started asking me questions about how come I was still in my pajamas and what was I doing out this time of day. I told him it was none of his business as long as he got paid, but first thing I knew he had turned around and came back here, pulled up out front, came in and got Miss Deming to come out and bring me in. I was so close to gettin' outta here. So close. I hate it. I can't stand it."

The burn kid, who most of the other patients in the ward thought was snooty and selfish, had tears in his eyes. There was no escape from the hospital, from the pain, from the scars that would pull at his skin and taunt him for as long as he lived. No hope for escape.

A few months later the morning maid was fired for sleeping on the job. A staffer found her sawing logs after she had come on duty. That same morning maid was teaching the ins and outs of moneylending to the Kid. Over a period of a couple of months the Kid had built a quarter up to four dollars. The maid first asked if she could borrow a quarter til payday, promising to pay him thirty cents. And again and again and again. Sixty cents for fifty. A dollar and a quarter for a dollar. The kid discovered the ecstasy of usury.

A couple of days before she was fired, he had lent the morning maid four dollars; she was going to give him five payday. She was fired two days before payday. She did not stop on her way from the bank to take care of that financial obligation. The Kid had a change of heart about prospects for his future fiscal well-being.

Those fifteen months passed so swiftly the Kid could hardly keep track. Peggy and Joe visited occasionally, most often when Joe Frankie got an assignment from ESSO to drive a wrecker to Memphis and Peggy would ride with him.

But they never came on Sunday. All the time the Kid was in the hospital he never had one visitor on a Sunday during regular visiting hours.

He was full of mischief, though, and could entertain himself by harassing folk and the sons and grandsons and nephews and brothers they were trying to see. The Kid was going to get attention somehow. Whatever it took. He was such a nuisance sometimes visitors wheeled their patient's bed down to the atrium or the auditorium for some peace and quiet, to get away from him. Polio hadn't changed his worrisome personality, all it did was make him more obnoxious for the lack of mobility.

Running his legs or running his mouth, the Kid was gonna be running something as long as he was breathing. The Kid was still running his mouth more than four decades later, still irritating folk with his semi-desperate attempts at humor and intelligence and philosophical insight.

When the visitors and visitees abandoned him, the Kid read. Miz Northcutt still came by every Friday morning with a new bundle of books and he read every one he could get his hands on. He read when he wasn't trying to get into mischief. He read during nap time when he could. Finally the aides, who had been coming over and grabbing his books from him, relented as long as he would be quiet and not let the young boys in the ward know what he was doing because they had to get their rest.

Crippled Children's geared a lot of activities toward challenging the intellect of their young charges. Reading abounded to stimulate lazy gray cells as well as to while away the boring hours between the pains of rehabilitation. Games of every ilk; the Kid played so much double deck canasta he tired of the game before he was discharged and never played it again for as long as he lived; and all the belts and wallets and paint-by-number pictures they made two hours at a time every afternoon from two til four.

The second time the Kid got the pinkeye it was an accident. They weren't threatening to send him home. He was having too good a time to be sick. Still, there it was. There were two of them. Larry, a kid not far from Paris, got it too. But Miss Mason wasn't about to give up her quarters this time. So the Kid and Larry got the little room with sliding doors across the hall from the dining room. I guess you could call it a utility room. Staff members used it for breaks and conferences and for taking unruly patients they were having trouble quieting down. There was barely room for the two hospital beds and no wiggle room, but it was one of the Kid's favorite places in the hospital.

Stay here until you're not contagious.

Sorry, boys, but orders is orders.

Sorry?

225

That was just about the best time the Kid had all the time he spent there and he had had hisself some good ole times. First, you could look out the window and down the way a bit and see the girls' ward. The Kid could see Nancy Rice, the love of his moment.

Aaah, Nancy, who'd sent him a photo of her standing by her bed holding the hem of her dress halfway up her thigh. Love, I tell you, conquers all other thoughts of all other things. And here he could see her and he just knew she'd show more skin for him before it was all said and done. She said she did. He said he saw it. Night after night.

Sad truth of the matter was, whether it was the pinkeye or poor eyesight or, more likely, poor angle, the boy couldn't see anything except some blurred movement once in awhile. The awful truth was that the best he could do was see her wave goodnight just before lights out. If she waved real big and vigorously.

But every day she sent a note to him via the girls' ward's aide: "Dear Kid. I dreamed about you again last night. Did you dream about me? I dreamed we were at the beach hugging and kissing and having so much fun. It was a wonderful dream, Kid. Did you see my show last night? The one just for you? Just before lights out? I hope you thought it was sexy because that's what I wanted you to think. I like you very much, Kid. Sometimes I wonder if I love you. Do you love me? Please destroy this note after you've read it. If you don't, we both will be in trouble."

Every movement in that window five hundred feet close during those few minutes before lights out every day was a sex show which he saw clearly in his mind as he commanded his eyes to see everything, to miss nothing, of the wonderful nekkid flesh of his beloved Nancy. And was sorely titillated.

The two patients in "isolation" were spoiled by staffers. The night aide for the girls' ward came down and played cards with 'em every night. The dietician, Miss Reily, from Ireland, came into the boys' room at least twice a day to say hi and tell a story about her childhood, always with a laugh. She was the primary spoiler; she gave those boys everything they wanted to eat.

Once the Kid complained to her about peanut butter and jelly sandwiches for supper. She went to the hospital director and suggested a change in the menu because the Kid was unhappy. If the Kid had known she was gonna do that, he'd a kept his trap shut. First thing he knows here comes the director into the little room. "The dietician tells me you don't like peanut butter and jelly. Is that right?" The Kid was too scared to say anything, so he didn't.

"All the food you eat is carefully planned because it's good for you patients. We are not going to change our menu for one or two patients, regardless of how long they have been here or how much members of the staff like them. Is that clear? There will be no favorites as long as I am here and I don't intend on leaving anytime soon. Do you understand that? Do we have a meeting of the minds on this matter which never should have come up in the first place?"

"Yes ma'am."

Minutes later Miss Reily came in with a couple of hamburgers for the Kid and Larry.

"I didn't know she'd go off halfcocked like that. Here. But don't tell anybody, you hear? Don't worry. You know I'll take care of you whenever I can."

One night the Kid had ELEVEN hamburgers. Ate so much he couldn't sleep for the bellyache, but it was one more than Larry. Showed that sumbitch up. Never give up. Never let go. Bulldogs ain't got nothin' on the Kid. Never did. Never will.

Which is one of the reasons he ran almost completely out of steam at age forty. One of the primary reasons he was forced to retreat from the real world and live in the dream world he created to save himself from self-destruction or dry rot or both. Or did he save himself? Was there ever any hope for him? Even in his type-A heyday? Or just some poor little fuck stuck in a motherless warp running around the wheel in his soul forever. A gerbil for whom the best possible outcome would be the surcease of forever forgetfulness.

Rehabilitation! But that's for another day. Another carp. Another sharp, incisive bombastic stinkbomb plopped splatteringly in the middle of Miss Manners' spotless living room floor, on that genuine, if almost imperceptibly blood-stained, polar bearskin rug.

The Kid pleaded with the night aide not to raise the side of his bed because it made him feel like a baby penned inside. Once in awhile they'd take pity on him and leave it down overnight.

One of those nights, back in the ward, he awoke in a shock of pain running rampant through his back like wildfire searing everything in its pathway. He had rolled out of bed and was hanging from the bars above his pillow. He remembered he had been dreaming about rolling over.

"Miss Deming! Miss Deming! Miss Deming!" He screamed the night aide's name over and over until, finally, there she was, bending over, lifting his feet back onto the bed just in time before he'd fallen completely down.

Although his back felt like it was still ablaze, he assured Miss Deming he was fine, that no damage had been done.

"Don't you go telling anybody I left your bars down, Kid. We'll both be in a lot of trouble if you do. Okay?"

"Yes ma'am. I won't tell."

"I'll get you some aspirin in case it starts to hurt after awhile. That way you can sleep."

Although his frantic calls for Miss Deming awakened other patients in the ward none of them ever told.

Not long after the Kid was released from the hospital, the Kid's back collapsed into serious scoliosis again. He would wonder the rest of his life whether falling out of bed that night contributed to his relapse. Because he had insisted that the side of his bed be left down. Because he didn't want to treated like a child.

The Kid's resentment of authority, nurtured by the flailing whips of Uncle Sam, reached adolescence in Crippled Children's Hospital where there was, again, no recourse, no appeal to orders he didn't like.

Which were practically all the orders.

Unfortunately for him and his mental health, he always forgot the special treatment he received from so many of the hospital personnel. All he could see was the color of anger at the helplessness he felt. *If they want to cut*

*me open alive, they can do it and I can't stop them. They give
me shots I can't stand. They give me mineral oil I don't want.
They give me orders I don't like. There is nothing they can't do
to me if they want to and there is nothing I can do to make them
quit.*

Grownups inflicting pain and then when he
"grew up" it was higher ups inflicting pain. Always the
certainty of helplessness. Nowhere to run to; nowhere to
hide. Didn't matter how hard he tried.

And so it was with each rejection, perceived as
well as actual, the Kid got for the rest of his life. No fucking idea on earth how to deal with being told he was ir-
relevant to the Universe. And not always able to conceal
his sense of helplessness beneath the facade of brash pro-
fanity.

And he always blushed at the slightest embarrassment, the first twinge of a guilty conscience, the tiniest
hint of conflagration with somebody. A red flag.

The shmoozing was supposed to be protection
against being boxed into corners where there was no out-
let. If he couldn't impress them with foul language and
his cockadoodle strut then he'd kiss their asses til they
turned around and gave him a smile.

Sometime near the middle of the afternoon, just
after nap time, near the middle of the summer of nineteen-fifty-six, the physical therapist pushed a wheelchair
into the ward and stopped at the side of the Kid's bed.

His old friend dread split through his guts. A jolt
of Black Death. He had been forewarned. Doctor Ingram
had assured him there was no reason for him not to go
home, that all he needed to do was to get on his feet and
he'd be home free in no time at all.

Nothing lasts forever.

Not even forever. Does it?

"Good news, Kid. Today you start learning to walk again. What is it? The third time? Or fourth? We can't let you go home until you build up your leg and foot strength and the doctor says he wants you out of here in three weeks. So here we go."

She lowered the side of his bed.

"Turn over on your stomach and slide down to the floor. I won't let anything happen. You won't fall. I promise you won't fall."

"There! Slowly. Slowly."

"You're standing! Your feet are tingling, aren't they? That's normal. Stand still for a minute or two and then we'll get you into the wheelchair and down to the therapy room."

"Okay?"

"I guess so." The Kid was trembling with the exertion of getting out of bed the first time in more than a year and from the fear of he didn't know what.

"Okay. Pick up your left foot and put it over here so we can get you into the wheelchair."

"Aaww!"

The Kid collapsed in pain against his bed, hanging on for dear life.

"What hurts?"

"My ankle. My ankle. I can't stand on it!"

On his first venture back to the world of walkers the Kid had sprained his ankle, delaying therapy for a week.

After which therapy came with a vengeance. His legs felt like they were being stuck full of pins until they got used to standing again, bit by bit. Then walking the parallel bars. Then walking. Without crutches for the first time since pre-Thanksgiving nineteen-fifty.

He was in PT every day, morning and afternoon. Tote that barge. Lift that bale. You fall down on your face and they'll send you to hell before they give you a break. Get up and move it, Kid. No slackers allowed inside that doorway, ya hear?

And he did. He still had to wear his steel-staved corset to keep him upright and his right leg was still pretty useless — he had to "sling it" from his hip — but he was walking without help and look at him go. The Kid suddenly saw that life for him was finally going to be normal. No more two hour naps every day. No more exercises morning and night. No more you can't do this and you can't do that because you're a poor little crippled boy. Hell, he could walk. There wudn't anything else to say, was there?

And, by god, the better he got at this walking thing, the more of a hurry he was to get back to grandmother's house, to a life outside the hospital. Until he could taste freedom from all the rules that had closely governed his life for nearly a year and a half.

By the time Peggy and Joe Frankie came for him that bright August morning he was packed and ready to ride. He could hardly sit still for the warden's instructions about what he could and couldn't do. That ten minutes seemed like an eternity. How many generations of mockingbirds had been born and died and reborn until they'd been transmogrified into disembodied voices mocking his physical prison while the warden was reeling off all that stuff.

Afterwards he made the rounds kissing and hugging all the pretty ones and all the other ones he could find, shaking hands and saying goodbye to the place that was home just before he rode out into the noonday sun up to U.S. 79. With nary a look back.

Yeah, there was that lonesome feeling down in the pit of his belly. He was going to miss the place and those people and the movies and all the pretty girls in a row, but he was too excited about getting back into the great big outdoors to be slowed down by that. He, after all, was riding to freedom.

Hallelujah! Praise Jesus!

Grandmother's house was strange looking. Strange feeling. Familiar but not. Alien but not. The feeling that swept over the Kid as Joe Frankie pulled into the graveled driveway was the deep sense of loneliness the Kid had gotten before whenever he returned to grandmother's from a trip.

Grandmother was there at the top of the porch steps waiting to give the Kid his welcome home hug. Jacky was out playing ball somewhere.

Peggy and Joe Frankie sat in rockers on the porch for a spell with grandmother and the Kid and then they were gone, leaving the Kid to swim alone. Or sink. The Kid got up and walked out onto the front yard to reacquaint himself with everything.

The Kid was in the front yard when Jacky came walking down, baseball glove and ball in hand, grinning that quirky grin of his.

"Hey, boy! You doin' okay?"

"Yeah."

"You sure now?"

"Yeah."

"Sorry I didn't get to come see you in Memphis, boy. Welcome back to the nuthouse, I guess. Same old shit here, Kid. She ain't changed a bit and I don't guess she ever will. I figger I'll just put up with her as long as I can and then do somethin else. Yeah, welcome back!"

The whole family who lived in Henry County straggled in over the next couple of weeks to greet their celebrity.

Ronald came up from the farm with Aunt Pearl and Uncle Ralph. Didn't say much. Ronald didn't ever say very much to the Kid. Just "hi." Then went off to huddle with Jacky. They were buddies. They could share physical activities, talk sports and stuff the Kid had not an inkling about.

Despite his year plus in Memphis the Kid soon found out he was still a less than perfect physical specimen. Still couldn't run. Still couldn't jump. Still couldn't stand up straight without his corset on. Jacky and Ronald had much more in common; when they got together the Kid understood that he was the audience, the wildly cheering crowd watching the game from the stands; that he would never be on the playing field although he would spend most of the rest of his life trying out for the team.

"You wanna come out and visit Ronald for a few days?" Aunt Pearl.

"Yes, please!" The Kid.

The farm was still the bastion of puredee pleasure it had been before for the Kid. Yepper, the Kid could have taken a lifetime of this.

It was cotton picking time. The Kid went out with Ronald to the patch and decided he'd try it. He must have worked for half an hour until he was too tired to stand up any longer and so retired to the grassy knoll at the side of the cotton patch.

That night lying in bed by the side of Ronald the Kid noticed his back felt different. It didn't exactly hurt, but it did feel "different". He reached back to his spine with his hand and felt a knot he hadn't noticed before. That is where it felt strange.

The Kid would never feel exactly the same again. He knew that night. He knew he'd fucked himself terribly and probably irreversibly. He never told anyone. He was too scared to tell anyone. Miserable. Didn't say anything. Hell, there wasn't anything to say. He'd fulfilled grandmother's Moody prophecy again. He had proved again he wasn't any good.

This time he had really proved it. To himself.

Welcome to the A & P

Being back in the general population was strange for the Kid. Adjusting to living outside the hospital was a tough as learning to walk all over again, except it took ever so much longer. As controlling as grandmother tried to be, she couldn't hold a candle to the rules and regulations of Crippled Children's. Nor did she have the staff to enforce them. Being at home was like being dropped in the middle of a big beautiful place without instructions on how to enjoy it. The Kid just kinda soaked it all up, blissfully enjoying the absence of the watchers.

Truth to tell, the Kid didn't know what to do with himself for most of the first year he was out of the hospital. It was like starving to death within reach of a magnificent buffet because everything was so good he couldn't make up his mind what to reach for first.

The Kid and Larry Grainger would go rambling through the woods behind Miz Bollus' house kicking through the thick blanket and looking for the thrill of the unknown and the unexpected. Larry Grainger would come to be his best friend in the whole wide world. Larry lived in the little block house up from Miz Bollus. Maybe they'd walk to Brockwell's Store and buy a Nehi raspberry with six cents from his secret hoard of cash. Maybe even add a nickel for a bag of salted peanuts and pour them into the cold drink because it was so good.

Or sit on the front porch where he had a front row seat on the theater that was the neighborhood with grandmother acting as the mistress of ceremonies introducing actual names and alleged events. Later, in the late fifties, grandmother would break down, make a desperate search for cash, find some, buy a television set, and become a stone soap opera addict. Before tv, however, grandmother saw Rorie Addition as a soap opera.

Life was so much looser on the outside, often discomfortingly so. The guidelines were vague compared to the hospitals. And there was all that spare time when the Kid didn't have to be anywhere. When he wasn't at school he followed Jacky around as much as he could. It would be months before the Kid felt truly comfortable in his new environment.

The fall of nineteen-fifty-six. Jacky began his sophomore year at E. W. Grove High School. Ronald started fifth grade at Puryear School. Peggy was in the early stages of her third year of marriage to Joe Frankie and the Kid was in the eighth grade at Atkins-Porter School.

Mister Loudy fancied himself to be a prize intimidator of eighth grade students, inflicting such serious pain on a thirteen or fourteen year old student in his homeroom as to be almost orgasmic for him.

Miz Ridgeway, the literature and English teacher, kept challenging the students. "Now if you can't do this work, just say calf rope." No one ever knew exactly what would happen if they said calf rope because nobody ever did.

The Kid didn't form any close friendships at school. He wasn't sure of his footing, or how to operate in an alien environment. These kids were dangling from strings wiggled by their testosterone and the Kid first of all didn't know that and second of all had no idea how to wield his influence with people his own age.

The Kid was regularly reminded of his poverty in any number of ways. His clothes were cheap and they looked it and he was keenly aware. He changed shirts on

Tuesdays and Thursdays. He wore the same pants all week long. He got his school lunches free until he got to high school where he carried his lunch with him.

He never had money to do things like all the other kids seemed to do. He wasn't all that sure what they did but he was sure it was something he'd enjoy the hell out of if he only had the money to do it.

Near the end of the school year Mister Loudy called him out of the room to tell him that the Paris Kiwanis Club had offered to buy his eighth grade graduation outfit. The Kid was both embarrassed and eager. He said he'd ask grandmother. She said yes.

A Kiwanian helped him pick out a light tan sport jacket with medium brown slacks to go with new shoes, socks, shirt and underwear. The Kid preened in those new threads. He looked like a regular kid. Good. Brand new flattop haircut Uncle Telous had given him — Uncle Telous was the family barber.

Brand new wardrobe, brand new haircut, he was ready for the world of quasi-psuedo matriculation. Eighth grade! Wheeeee!

His childhood was over now. High school in the fall heralded entry into the magical kingdom of betterness. The Kid knew for certain from now on he'd always be better than those grade schoolers. 'Cause he was grown up. Had the certificate to prove it. Jumping from the kiddy pool to the deep end of the big 'un over there. He was ripe for it. *Watch out, girls, here I come. Ye can't git away now. I gotcha. And if I ain't gotcha, I'm gonna getcha. You betcha. Hell yes!*

During the summer of nineteen-fifty-seven the Kid celebrated the rite of that passage.

He did have some sho' nuf fun. Damn! True and sure. Two — count 'em — two adventure vacations. Plus the weeks of palling around with Larry Grainger, his by-now-by-god best buddy. Two weeks of running wild and being free to get into all the trouble he could stand in St. Louis, the Gateway to the West, and to pleasure himself endlessly. Then two more weeks with Peggy and Joe Frankie and the kids in Louisville "running the streets", looking for little bitty women without any clothes on while he was selling religious placards.

Had those trips not come up the Kid would still have been as happy as a bug in a rug. Larry and he gallivanted all over the land, exploring and experimenting and learning stuff. Larry taught the Kid many things, perhaps most importantly, the facts of life as they would have been in a perfect world, which is what it was during those halcyon days.

The Kid would have exhausted himself putting killer moves on the ladies after that, would have kissed half the girls in Rorie Addition half to death as he waltzed around in his newfound knowledge of the secret life of men and women under the rosebush and sundry other coverings. If he hadn't been so shy.

He was so shy he could hardly bring himself to say hello to a girl, much less suggest adventures that would inevitably wind up making whoopee as he knew they must because Larry had given him the skinny. Oh, his face would turn bright red and his toes would curl up in defense against the...the...whatever the hell it was that would grab him and gobble him down, clothes and all, if he spoke up in front of any female he came across.

That's the only part Larry couldn't help him with. How to get past the barrier of shy so he could get down to business.

Miz Bollus' son Leonard drove the Kid up to his house in suburban St. Louis for two weeks. Leonard lived with his wife and two stepchildren; a boy, Raymond, who was a year or two older than the Kid and a girl, Marilyn, who was a year or two younger.

During his two weeks there, he saw Raymond and Marilyn do whatever they wanted to do whenever they wanted to do it. If they needed transportation their mom hopped in the car and drove them there. No questions asked. No fuss, no muss, no yelling, no screaming.

Mrs. Bollus spent hardly any time in the kitchen. The family thrived on junk food and quick food and whatever they wanted to eat. The Kid thought he had died and gone to heaven when he learned he could have baloney sandwiches every single day he was in St. Louis if he wanted them.

No sweat.

With *mayo* which he knew meant they were rich, else how could they afford mayonnaise at every meal if they wanted it?

The Kid was about five foot eight that summer. Or at least he had been back when Mister Loudy measured everybody in class the previous year. Raymond was a head taller and heavier. A little on the stout side, keeping himself out of fat by running around all the time. The Kid often could hardly keep up with him on their jaunts about suburbia that summer.

Raymond and the Kid quickly became ace-boon-coons. It was like they had known each other all their lives. Partners in crime. Partners in adventure. Partners in summer vacationing. Whatever one would suggest the other would agree to. Not one argument in two weeks. Not one.

One of their favorite things to do, when they weren't out wandering through the neighborhoods talking about important stuff or sitting in the living room watching old movies on television and swilling cold drinks, was chemistry. In its old sense, that is. Mixing different chemical compounds in a test tube and see what happens. They tried to make explosives, although neither had offered any idea what to do with the stuff or what they were doing. It was a time of experimentation.

The pair worked on chemical experiments every day, using the Kid's host's chemistry set. When they ran out of chemicals, they'd put an empty detergent box in a shopping bag, walk up to the neighborhood drugstore and steal more. The Kid never was sure why they stole the alarm clock which was never used, or intended to be used, as a part of a chemistry experiment.

And at the end of the two weeks it still wasn't over! Mrs. Bollus, on the afternoon before they were to leave for Paris, asked the Kid to go to the mall with her, just the two of them. When they got to the mall, he walked with her into a big department store and stopped at boy's clothes. "I've been thinking about a going away present for you," she said. "Would you be insulted if Leonard and I bought you some clothes to wear to school this fall?"

"No ma'am." Pants and shirts and underwear and socks!

Lemme never wake up from this dream. For two weeks in the summer of fifty-seven.

A Rodman Court Excursion

"Hey, boy! You forgit somethin?"

"Hey, you! I'm talkin' to you!"

"Stop if you know what's good for you!"

Busted!

Fear froze the Kid. He couldn't run. God had seen to that with a little polio whiplash effect. Hell, he couldn't move. He'd just walked out of a Kroger store in Louisville, Kentucky with contraband hidden under his shirt. He'd stolen a pack of cigarettes and two bars of candy. And walked out, heady with the success of his foul deed.

"Now come back over here, boy. Come here. Right now!"

The Kid slowly turned to face life at hard labor. Or worse, that they would tell Peggy and Peggy would tell grandmother and grandmother would tell everybody she knew or whose telephone number she knew and the Kid would be in disgrace. Again.

Why? Why? Why'd I do it? Why? Why?

He hoped he'd die before he got back to the guy who, by now, was backed up by a woman in a Kroger clerk uniform, the same woman he'd bought one piece of candy from so she wouldn't know he'd stole the rest.

"Did you forgit to pay for a pack of cigarettes, boy? Or did you steal 'em? This lady here says you left without paying? Is that true? Do you think we should call the police or your family? Speak up, boy!"

"I forgot to pay, sir. I have the money right here."

The Kid pulled a dollar bill out of his pants pocket and handed it to the guy dressed in a blue Kroger smock, quaking. If they knew about everything he'd stolen he wouldn't be able to pay for it and it'd be curtains for sure and certain.

The guy grabbed the bill, then dug into his pants pocket.

"Here's your change. If I's you I'd find someplace else to shop without paying. Or better still, I think I'd give it up altogether. You'll just be caught and eventually you know you're gonna be arrested. That's good advice, boy. Good advice to take while there's still time for it to do you some good."

"You can go now."

The Kid was so weak he could hardly stand. He stumbled over to a nearby fire hydrant and leaned against it. Scared shitless and heaving sighs of relief at the same time. He'd pushed it to the edge again. And fallen over. And he was still alive. *And I'm gonna stay this way. No more stealin'. Never again. It's not worth it. I almost went to jail! They coulda told everybody I know. I couldn't have faced anybody ever again! I'm quittin' this stuff. Today. Right now!*

The Kid spent much of his summer vacation in Louisville walking, exploring the limits of the legs which a year previously had been propped up in a hospital bed, useless as teats on a boar hog. Sitting inside the Rodman Avenue apartment got real close real often, so his walkabouts were welcome relief to both Peggy and him. Once he was outside the front door of Peggy's apartment he was on his own.

Street after street of low and middle income housing. In every direction it looked like a lot of people didn't care a lot about how their houses and their yards looked. Total exhilaration for a minute and then scary as hell. He had no limit to his meanderings yet at the same time was overwhelmed by the feeling that he was completely isolated in a strange place and at the mercy of whoever wanted to do whatever to him.

This was the year the Kid went into business for himself. In Paris he'd sent off for decorative biblical plaques to sell, knowing he was smart enough and ambitious enough to make his fortune.

To the door.

Knocking.

Knocking.

"Are you selling something?"

"Yes ma'am. These religious plaques. They're just fifty cents apiece and they would look real nice on your living or bedroom walls."

"Well, we don't want any."

As she turned around to herd her little duo back into the black maw of her home the Kid saw — or thought he saw — that she was clad only in her underwear.

It was about then that a light went off in his head.

If I knock on enough doors some lady is going to open it up nekkid. She won't have any clothes on.

It was a sign from the god of pubescence.

It was a motivating sign.

The Kid vowed he would not stop knocking on doors until one was answered by a nekkid lady and he knew what would happen then, just as sure as he could be.

He was ecstatic.

Not that anybody paid any attention to the Kid's sales pitch except for the dozen or so who were dumber than his pitch and couldn't endure the sound of that little bit of loose change rattling around in their cracked cookie jars. He had been lucky to sell one or two a day, but was disappointed that none of those good-looking ladies invited him in for tea and sex. Or the kinda good-looking ones. Hell, not even a single one of even the ugliest women he'd ever seen in his life. He was sorely disappointed on many fronts. Couldn't make any money and couldn't get laid.

Not even anymore in their underwear until a year later when Kay Oliver answered the door when he and Larry went up to sell some greeting cards in Paris. She was the picture of modesty, poking her head out the door holding on for dear life. Until the Kid saw the reflection of the rest of her in the full length mirror three feet behind her on the back wall of the foyer.

It might accurately be said of the Kid that summer that he was obsessed with bare skin of the feminine variety. His search for nekkid women was never-ending.

One bright and sunny day, while Peggy and Joe Frankie were shopping in some exotic place of business in the Louisville environs and the Kid was waiting in the Ford, he made one of his random, but regular, searches. Looking. Just looking. He'd take whatever he got. If there wasn't anything to take, maybe there'd be something to see.

The Kid laid down on the back seat and stuck his head down so he'd get a good look at anything interesting under the front seat. It looked like there was something under Joe Frankie's side! The Kid reached under and pulled out a magazine. Bingo!

His heart started pounding. His face burned like fire. His search for nekkid women had paid off! Kinda. A skin magazine. Filled with unclothed women in erotic poses. Page after page of wonders like the Kid had never seen before. So this is what Aunt Naomi was trying to hide when she chased him out of the kitchen! And all of those other women who got pissed off when he tried to take a peek at what was under their clothes.

Glory! Glory! Glory!

Something made the Kid look up to see Peggy and Joe Frankie walking across the parking lot to the car. He quickly shoved the magazine back under the seat and commenced to compose himself so nobody could tell he'd just seen one of the two or three wonders of the world.

They didn't say a thing. They didn't suspect a thing.

It was cool!

But not enough. The Kid wanted to see more of those pictures. He waited until there was nobody about the car for his heist. Soon the magazine was safely ensconced in the back of the closet in Peggy's bathroom.

Semper Paratus!

Until the day the Kid's attention was rudely diverted from the television set he and Sandra, the first born, were watching.

"Kid, come here!"

A bomb exploded in the Kid's head. Psychic or not, he knew exactly what had happened. Instantly. As his heart sank, he again wished himself out of existence to somewhere else. To anywhere else. *Oh, God! I've done it again. Oh, God! What's gonna happen to me? What's she gonna do?* He knew that in a few minutes he'd be plummeting down a black hole to what he knew must be hell, holding a ticket issued by his sister.

"Where'd you get this?" Peggy was holding the magazine in her hand as she scowled at her younger brother.

"It's not mine."

"This was in Joe Frankie's car and he says he didn't bring it in the house, so you must have."

"I don't know where it came from."

"Well, regardless of where it came from, you keep your hands off stuff that is not yours. Do you understand?"

The Kid nodded his head semi-vigorously.

"And I mean it, Kid."

The Kid's head nodded faster, ever faster.

"That's all then. I don't want to have to talk to you about this again."

Relief. He hadn't died. Life was possible after disclosure of his recent criminal past. The magazine disappeared from the bathroom closet. Nobody mentioned it to the Kid anymore. And, after a couple of days, Peggy didn't seem to be holding a grudge.

Life resumed.

Peggy washed her family's clothes in a wringer washer. She hung her clothes out to dry in back of their apartment.

One morning as the Kid was eating his cereal at the dining table four or five feet in front of the washer, he heard a scream and looked up to see Peggy's hand coming through the wringer! Then her wrist and her arm! Almost up to the elbow. As Peggy turned white with pain and panic, the Kid couldn't move. Did not move to help his sister. Could not have if he had known, or remembered, what to do.

It looked like Peggy's arm was going to be pulled out of her shoulder. Just as the rollers pulled the arm up to the elbow, Peggy somehow found the presence of mind to hit the release bar which caused the rollers to jump apart and allowed her to extricate her arm which had been pressed flat way up past her wrist.

"Kid, go get the neighbor lady. Tell her what happened and that I need her."

Peggy was white with pain, but stoic.

The Kid raced to summon the neighbor. He stayed with the kids while the neighbor drove her to the hospital, her arm just sorta hanging limply at her side. She might be gone for days. Weeks even as bad as it looked like she was hurt.

But she wasn't. They were back within a couple of hours. No serious injuries.

The next week the Kid went back to Tennessee.

The Kid never felt more welcome anywhere in his life than he did when he walked into that crummy little concrete block home.

The Graingers lived in the same house where Tommy Fox and his mom had lived.

Dirty white on the outside, plopped down in the middle of a patch of mostly bare dirt or mud, depending on current weather conditions. Dark and damp and musty on the inside. A living room, kitchen, and two bedrooms.

The Kid was at Larry's house just about every day. It was like having a real family. They didn't pay any more attention to him than they did their own. He became one of them and that became his addiction.

What the Kid found in that dingy house with no indoor plumbing and very little else in the way of human comfort was love and laughter. What he found was sanctuary. A place where he felt happy and safe and protected against the sticks and stones that hurdled with bone-breaking acuity through the air beyond the safety zone.

Larry's dad, Dalton, was mostly unemployed for the first couple of years the Kid and Larry were friends. He didn't spend much time around the house, though, and the Kid was glad for that because he found him to be too threatening, too much a reminder of Uncle Sam.

His brother and he raised goats out at Cottage Grove and sold their meat door to door. That was probably the tip of the iceberg of their homemade enterprise, but that was all the Kid saw ever over the years. Actually,

Mr. Grainger was a fireman for the L&N Railroad and had been laid off.

The Kid first met Larry Grainger up by Miz Bollus' front porch. There was no doubt that Larry, like the Kid, was a denizen of poor, southern white America. Slender, freckled face. A big cowlick over his right eye and an Elvis-style permanent sneer snaking up the right side of his upper lip, giving his mouth the look of something between Elvis and Ricky Nelson.

But Larry couldn't sing. Larry couldn't read very well. There wasn't a whole lot Larry was good at. Except having a good time.

And knowing everything exciting there was to know about life.

And knowing everything there was to know about girls.

And knowing how to teach some of his multiple talents to the Kid.

The Kid was a dreamer; he spent years reading and exploring the terrain of his vivid imagination. He dreamt about adventures; Larry had adventures.

He dreamt about women; Larry lost his cherry at twelve or thirteen.

Larry Grainger became the Kid's real world teacher.

Every day spent with Larry was to the Kid an exciting classroom. Larry taught him how to smoke. He had never even heard about masturbation until Larry told him about it. If it hadn't been for Larry Grainger, the Kid never would have learned to ride a bicycle.

Having adventures was Larry's specialty and he generously shared his expertise with the Kid as the two of them happily roamed the woods and railroad tracks and back roads and bottomlands of west Paris.

The relationship between the Kid and Larry grew rapidly. For the first weeks the Kid didn't go into Larry's house. They'd meet at the Kid's house and walk into the woods or the Kid would go up to the Grainger's house to play baseball at the end of their kinda gravelled driveway.

The baseball was what brought sheer fun into the Kid's life for the first time since Jacky and he had played with their old car tires on the road and in the gullies down by the old log house in Whitlock. There wasn't much talent on the team which played against itself, but it wasn't from a lack of effort. Linda, Larry's sister, would scrunch up her eyes and run like a fullback chasing a ball or a runner, as if her life depended on it. They played with ferocity that summer with other kids from the neighborhood, using up the last iota of energy to get a hit or an out, draining themselves totally in the name of having fun in that old front yard.

Whoever taught Larry to have fun did a real good job. The laughs, however, didn't last long enough. When he was thirty and change, Larry's body was found hanging in a cell of the Henry County Jail. Suicide the cops said. "Suicide, hell!" Linda said. "I heard they's beatin' hell out of him before they ever put him in that squad car to take him to jail. I don't believe for a minute it was suicide. 'Course now I can't prove it and can't nobody else neither. You know Larry. As contrary as the day was long. I think he pissed off one person too many and got hisself killed for it."

Scarcely more than a decade after he opened the door to all those wonderful adventures for the Kid he was senselessly dead. By his own hand or someone else's, a stunning explosion of reality for the Kid who'd deferred to the greater knowledge and skill of the younger man to his heart's delight. Time after time.

Larry had an old beat up bike that one or the other of the kids was always riding around the house. So much so that the bicycle had worn off all the grass, leaving a dirt track.

"You ever ride a bicycle, Kid?"

"Nope."

"Ever want to?"

"Yeah. Lots of times."

"Well, git on this here thang and I'll hold ye up and you can get yerself a ride."

"I don't know."

"Hell, what's the worst thang that can happen? You'd fall off, right? And that's no big deal. And it ain't likely to happen long's I'm holdin' on to the bike. Come on."

"Well. Okay."

Kerplop! Halfway around the house the bicycle, the Kid and Larry slammed to the ground ass-over-tea-kettle.

"See that didn't hurt did it? That's all the bad it hurts iffen you fall."

"Yeah, that's not bad at all," answered the Kid who, in reality, was holding back the part about his back

252

and rib cage feeling like he'd been dropped from an airplane without a parachute. Hurt like a motherfucker, but damned if he was going to say anything about that! What! And be a sissy?

"Wanna do it again?"

"Okay."

"Hang on there. Hang on."

The Kid had all the balance of a side of beef. He leaned too far and sent them all to the ground again.

"Ye gotta try to get yer balance next time, Kid. That's what ye need to ride a bicycle. And not much else. Hell, if ye can peddle the damn thing, ye can ride it, once ye've got yer balance."

"Let's go again."

A week of practice went by.

The Kid was thankful the bruises he incurred from the ravages of training were mostly under clothes and away from the prying eyes of grandmother.

And then one day he rode that damned bicycle!

By himself.

All the way around the Grainger house.

And felt the breeze from the speed breathe a new thrill of accomplishment into his being.

Grandmother eventually found out that the Kid had gone and learned to ride a bike. She had little to say about it, uncharacteristically. Perhaps, the Kid thought, because it was a fait accompli.

After he learned to ride, the Kid would ride the bike down the road and Larry would run alongside.

When the Graingers had a second bike for the girls for a little while before it broke down permanently, the Kid and Larry would explore the world of Rorie Addition together. Nothing finer than pedaling down the road with your best pal smack dab into the middle of life filled with never ending excitement.

For three years or more the Kid and Larry were inseparable like a pubescent two-headed monster. Seemed like, when the Kid didn't have chores, they were always together, cooking up some fantasy or the other and spending an awful lot of energy turning those fantasies into reality. They talked about adventures as they sat in the Grainger living room smoking their cigarettes, savoring the unscarred vitality of kids not yet shackled by cynicism.

The boys had to find a place to conceal themselves from the prying eyes of the outside world — outside defined as anybody besides the two compadres. And they did. Not thirty feet from Larry's house was the perfect spot. Special made, it seemed, to fit two burgeoning adventurers. Course all it really was was a middlin' sized depression in a mound of grassy dirt, but for the rest of their relationship that's where they'd go to confer about the sacred and the secret. And even the commonplace.

It was in that spot that the Kid first hypnotized Larry, a trick he had read about in a library book. "Close your eyes and relax. Pretend you're in a tall building. On an elevator at the top floor. There are ten floors. As you pass each floor you will relax more, become more comfortable and find your mind moving toward a greater peace than it has ever known."

"Just relax as the elevator goes down."

"You're passing the ninth floor now. You can already feel the peace beginning to cover you like a warm and cuddly blanket."

Until they got to the first floor when the Kid assured Larry that he was totally relaxed, fast asleep and ready for any instruction the Kid had for him.

Larry's eyes were closed and the Kid thought he looked pretty relaxed.

"Open your eyes."

Larry's eyelids slowly parted. His eyes looked kinda dead to the Kid. Didn't seem to show any emotion or anything else. They were just open.

"Bark like a dog," commanded the Kid.

"Arf!"

"Arf!"

The book says if he's really hypnotized he'll bark. That don't sound like a bark. He could do better than that if he wasn't hypnotized.

"Larry, I want you to pay attention to me now. I'm going to light this match and then I'm going to hold this burning match under your finger. When I do you won't feel a thing."

"Do you understand?"

"Yes."

"Hold your hand over here. Palms down."

The Kid struck the match on the side of its box, let it flare, then moved it to half an inch under Larry's right index finger.

He watched Larry's face closely.

Larry didn't flinch.

Nothing.

The Kid held the flame until the match was totally consumed, except for the last little part that he needed to hang onto so the Kid didn't burn his own damn self.

There was no sign of a reaction from Larry.

"Turn your hand over."

There was no sign of a burn on Larry's finger.

Nothing.

"Okay, Larry, we're going to bring you out of your trance now. When I count to three and snap my fingers, you'll wake up refreshed and feeling wonderful. You won't remember anything that happened. And your finger will not be affected by the match in any way."

"Do you understand?"

"Yes."

"Okay." "One." "Two." "Three."

Snap!

"Now you're awake, aren't you?"

"Yep."

"How ya feel?" "Do you feel anything, like pain?"

"No. Not even a little bit."

Having completed their secret business of the day, the pair got up and walked into Larry's house where they lit up a couple of cigarettes in the living room to talk about what they'd just done. Within fifteen minutes of coming in, the entire outer joint of Larry's right forefinger blew up into a single gigantic blister. Almost as if he'd pressed it against a hot wood cookstove (or got burnt by a match in a mysterious amateur hypnotizing incident).

Larry never could be hypnotized after that, in spite of the Kid's best efforts. Which were awesome. And many.

At the Kid's request, Larry hypnotized him once in grandmother's house while she was out visiting. And told the Kid he could walk up and down stairs normally instead of climbing with his left leg and then lifting his right foot to that step. Slowly and awkwardly. More than just about anything else in the world the Kid wanted to be physically normal.

It didn't feel like Larry was doing such a hot job, although he did go through all the motions the Kid had taught him.

Afterwards the Kid didn't notice any difference.

Until Monday morning.

At school.

When, for the first time since November of nineteen-fifty, he walked up the steps to Grove High School normally. One foot up, the other foot to the next. No foot waiting on the other foot. No dragging.

There would be few moments in the Kid's life as delicious as that.

For two whole days.

On the third day it didn't work anymore. And it never worked again.

One healing miracle didn't go awry for the Kid. During his prepubescent years he was plagued with warts on his fingers. Accursed warts! It seemed like no matter what the Kid was grabbing for, the warts sped to the epicenter of his grasp and ran interference.

He pulled them off, they grew back.

How he hated those monstrosities growing and seeding and spreading like the plague they were.

Larry's mom sympathized. "Ye know, Dalton's brother can git rid of them there thangs. He's got the gift for a fact. He's removed I don't know how many of 'em for me and the kids. Next time he's up 'ere if ye'll remind me I'll have him take a look."

Later Miz Grainger remembered. "Why 'on't ye take a look at the warts on this boy's hand? See if ye c'n git rid of 'em."

"Come here, boy. Stand right here. Hand me that hand with the warts on it." The other Mister Grainger looked at the Kid's hand, rubbed the warts lightly and released the hand.

"Now, iffen you won't look at them warts, they'll be gone in three weeks. But iffen ye look at 'em they won't go away. Understand?"

"Yessir."

As he walked out of the house with Larry, Larry said, "most times I seen him do it, he didn't do it that way. But I reckon it works mostly. I never seen it not work anyhow."

Having determined he would not look at his left hand, no matter what, for the next three weeks the Kid's eyes were drawn to his left hand but he didn't look.

Day after day, he'd go into the bathroom and start to look at his hands when he soaped them up and suddenly remembered. Just in time.

Three weeks later, to the day, the Kid held up his left hand to his eyes. The warts were gone!

They never did come back.

So how can a middle-aged man rubbing his dirty fingers across a snot-nosed kid's fingers get rid of the nuisance of warts whose geneses is a virus?

The Kid had gotten a chemistry set from kids up the street not long after he came home from his trip to St. Louis where, among other things, Raymond had excited his interest in mixing stuff together to see how chemicals reacted with each other.

There wasn't much to see in the real world, but in the rich recesses of his fertile mind the Kid was a mad scientist standing over a hot Bunsen burner developing the elixir of life. Or, driven by the curiosity that had consumed him his whole life, he simply wanted to see what would happen when he mixed things together. Even before the chemistry set.

With it, he felt like a wizard. Hell, he could make colors change, create solids out of liquids, do all kinds of neat things. There was no end to the magic he could work. Out in the shop side of the chicken coop Larry and he spent a lot of time there one summer, working the chemicals. Away from the prying eyes of adults.

The Kid graduated from not selling religious plaques to not selling Cloverine Salve. Always looking for a way around grandmother's, "I ain't got no money, Kid. I ain't got a cent I can spare beyond what it costs to raise you kids."

An ad in a comic book brought him his package of Cloverine Salve. Good for burns and minor wounds and for soothing the skin. He also sent off for greeting cards. So now he could fail in two major efforts simultaneously.

Once his chores were finished on Saturday morning, he'd strike out, often with Larry in tow. Miz Grainger wouldn't let Larry get a job while he was a kid. Said it was his father's job to support the family and that she wouldn't have no "kid of mine workin' when the daddy's got that responsibility."

While the Kid's finances never did improve much, the Grainger's did. Once Mister Grainger went back to work on the railroad, money was rolling in. So it seemed.

There was suddenly money for clothes and pop and taking trips in the forty-nine or fifty Cadillac Mr. Grainger bought. Worst of all, spending more time away from home. And the Kid.

Still there was time for some occasional fun.

Like the night the two killed one of Miz Grainger's chickens to satisfy their craving for fried chicken. Larry said he knew how to fry it. They plucked it, gutted it, cut it up and threw it in some flour. Thence into the skillet.

About that time the rest of the Grainger's made a sudden return from one of those side trips.

"I think they're back!"

"Quick, put that flour up and dump the chicken out of the skillet. Maybe Momma won't see anything wrong."

"I'll put the chicken in this bag."

"Let's get outta here so they won't know we've been here."

They took the raw chicken out back down into the woods and gnawed on a couple of pieces before they agreed they'd shown sufficient machismo to toss the rest to the dogs.

Tell the truth, they agreed it wudn't all that good raw.

The Other Brother Bites the Dust

There may have been some truth in Jacky's belief that he was the worst treated among the Moody kids by grandmother.

Ronald left her house at the age of six and so was, in her mind, a sweet innocent child. Up to her dying day she wondered why he never came to see her.

Peggy was a girl and got the kind of preferential treatment grandmother naturally afforded a girl, although Peggy herself never thought her treatment there was especially preferential. Ask her and if she were in an expansive mood she would recite the long litany of wrongs perpetrated against her physically, socially and emotionally.

The Kid had the sympathy vote from his polio, which he needed real bad because the consensus was he was the real asshole among the bunch.

That left Jacky to be the whipping boy. Not that he was whipped that much, but he was targeted for emotional mistreatment. Physical beating would not have brutalized his soul as much.

Jacky was pretty much a stranger to the Kid when he came back home from Memphis. Neither grandmother nor Jacky had visited him during his more than fifteen months in the hospital and both of them looked, and felt, pretty alien for awhile.

Despite all the blowhard bullshit that often made him look like a raging bull, the generous soul of Jacky — the inner core that the Kid was one of the few privy to — was soft and loving. He had to keep that part private from most folks. Folks who were more than able to use it to hurt him.

Before and after the Kid got home, Jacky stayed away from grandmother's as much as he could, finding any kind of sports activity as an excuse. He apologized to the Kid. "I'm sorry bro, but I jes' can't stand that woman. I hope you understand. It's got nothin' to do with you and everything to do with her. No matter what I do, it ain't enough to satisfy her. We're okay, aren't we?"

"You and me? Sure."

"You sure now?"

"Sure."

He had a heart as big as all outdoors. When they slept in the same bed during the days of his paper carrying, almost every night Jacky would have a big chocolate bar he'd share with the Kid under the covers. (Until he got fired because he threw away his papers instead of delivering them so he could play ball when he was supposed to be working.)

Until sometime after he went into the Army he couldn't bear to see any living thing hurt. A big softy who never learned to take care of himself, perhaps because nobody ever taught him to take care of himself, even though grandmother and others would vehemently disagree with that.

Jacky was self-appointed protector of the Kid. At school. At home. No matter how much they fought each other — and they fought each other a helluva lot (mostly when the Kid attacked Jacky) — you had to get through Jacky to get to the Kid and there weren't many folks, old or young, who could, or did, manage it.

263

They didn't seem to engage in many "brotherly" type activities, mostly, he figured, because Jacky's pleasures, outside of eating, came from sports, physically active sports, an area from which the Kid was effectively excluded, however vehemently he railed against his physical limitations by words and by playing baseball and hide-and-seek and kick-the-can.

Jacky loved to play football. Although it was a head injury that aborted his football career in college, in high school he thought, and played like, he was invincible. Undoubtedly, the most success Jacky ever found in life was on the high school football field and the most happiness on the field or the baseball diamond.

Still, there was a close bond shared by the two brothers. A love that reached far beyond their Moody egos and mule headedness. One thing the two shared was a passion for reading. It drove grandmother crazy. Two kids wasting all that time lookin' at books when they could have been working or doing something constructive.

Grandmother never seemed to let up on Jacky. It wasn't so much that her carping got worse as that it had a cumulative effect. Like varnish. Or arsenic.

The Kid and grandmother had just finished eating supper which featured baked sweet potatoes. The Kid was still sitting at the table, his head leaning on his hands propped on the tabletop.

Jacky's heavy footsteps clumped on the tired back porch.

Bang! The screen door slammed.

"Hey!" Jacky to the Kid.

"Hey!" the Kid to Jacky.

"What's there to eat in here?"

Grandmother, who was sitting on the couch in the living room, looked up. "There's some sweet taters in the frigerator. They should still be warm. Yer plate's set."

Jacky opened the refrigerator door, bent over and took out the sweet potatoes and a stick of butter, sat down, put a sweet potato on his plate and reached over to get the butter just as grandmother popped in the doorway. "Don't eat all that butter, Jacky. I ain't got no more and that's gotta last. I know you and you'll take it all if I don't say somethin'."

The wrong words on the wrong day to the wrong person.

As if all the wrongs against him had come together to savage him once again after he'd reached the absolute limit of being fucked, Jacky jumped to his feet.

"I don't want yer damned butter!"

Opened the refrigerator door and threw the stick of butter into its interior, spewing it all over the insides. Slammed the refrigerator door with such force that it rocked on its teeny little metal legs with the big round flat feet.

Stomped into the back bedroom — his bedroom — and started throwing clothes into a paper grocery bag.

"What in the world are ye doing, Jack?" asked grandmother, perplexed.

"I'm gettin' outta here! Somethin' I shoulda done a long time ago. Maybe now you can find your damned peace. And maybe give the Kid some of it."

Tears flowed. Voice broke. "All I asked you do, son, was not use all the butter. I don't know how I could have asked any nicer."

No response.

Jacky continued to sling articles of clothing, shaving gear and other stuff into the bag. "I'm gone!" he growled loudly. "Kid, this has nothing to do with you. I want you to know that. It has everything to do with her." He nodded toward the living room to which grandmother had returned with her tears.

And he left grandmother's house. Forever, at age seventeen.

First to the Paris Fire Department where the firemen gave him a bunk upstairs in the firehouse downtown.

Thence to the semi-palatial home of Harold Jackson, bigwig at the Carburetor Plant, where he stayed for as long as he could take it.

Jacky worked his way through the rest of high school. Although in some ways he was more alone than he had been at grandmother's, in other ways it looked like he wasn't nearly as alone as he had been at grandmother's.

Life seemed to pick him up and carry him along on its shoulders between there and high school graduation.

And by gosh and by golly, Jacky did graduate from E. W. Grove High School in Paris in the spring of nineteen-fifty-nine. And he did get a football scholarship to Murray State College twenty miles up the road in Murray, Kentucky.

And he did get kicked in the head the first week of practice. Hard enough to scare Jacky enough to drop out of football, to drop out of college and to join the US Army where he spent the next eight years of his life.

The Runaways

The evening air was like it always is, mostly, on an early summer evening in Henry County, Tennessee; darkening.

"Can I ride your bike home if I bring it back to-morrow?" The Kid.

"Why shore!" Larry Grainger.

And away he goes. Like the wind. After months of practicing, he's finally ready to let grandmother see him ride, knowing that when she sees how good he is she won't have, *can't* have, any arguments about his being hurt or killed or protests that she can't afford neither a doctor nor a funeral and that "y'alls money done run out long ago."

Down the Grainger driveway to the street. Left. Slowing down in front of Miz Bollus' house in prepara-tion for the big turn. A sweeping left turn into grand-mother's driveway. Grin a country mile wide on his face. She's never actually seen him ride before, that he knew of. Over the culvert. Grandmother's ho!

But wait! Something's gone wrong. The damn thang ain't turning. Before the Kid could much start thinking about what he was doing wrong, POW! Smack dab into the fork of the locust tree downhill from the driveway.

KERSPLAT! Ass-over-teakettle, the Kid was cata-pulted to the ground, and a grand show it was. For an audience of one. Grandmother.

"Kid if I've told you once I've told you a thousand times to stay off that bicycle. Ye jes' ain't able to do it. No telling what you've done to yer back now."

The Kid shook the grogginess in his head away, got up on his knees and felt the impact of a ball-peen hammer deep in the middle of his back. It hurt. A lot!

Jesus! But I won't give you the satisfaction of knowing I hurt myself, old woman. Nobody'll ever know but me. Get up now and act like it was nothing, nothing at all. Come on, Kid, git yer ass up if you don't want her thinking you really are some kind of cripple.

"Are ye hurt? Ye ain't gettin' up very fast."

"I'm okay. Dudn't look like I hurt anything, at least that I can tell."

The Kid pushed himself to his feet with his arms and, compensating for the weakness in his right leg, grabbed one fork of the locust tree and pulled himself straight to view the damage.

Dudn't look like the bike's hurt. Bent over and pulled it up off the ground and pushed it to the side of the house where he leaned it before walking up to the porch.

"I'm tellin' ye now fer the last time, Kid, don't ever let me catch you ridin' a bicycle again. Ye can't do it and I won't have it. And I won't have ye sneaking around behind my back to do it, either."

"Ye hear me, boy?"

"Yes ma'am."

"No more bicycle. That's it!"

As the Kid stood there in front of her he tried desperately to wish his grandmother into another dimension. He managed to keep a lid on his mouth but his temper hammered down and clanged the carnival bell. All the way to the top!

Who does she think she is? I'll show her. I don't have to take this stuff. I never wanted to live here in the first place. All I did was ride a bicycle.

You'd think from the way she's carrying on that I robbed a bank or killed somebody. What's she want from me? Whatever it is I ain't got it no more.

Why can't I have a home like Ronald? Aunt Pearl and Uncle Ralph would be laughing and stuff now. They wouldn't be bitching.

Ronald can do anything his little heart desires. He can have all the fun he can think of and all I get is grandmother who ain't gonna let me have any fun if she can help it.

All I get is fussed at. I wonder what they'd do if I wuz to jes' show up at their house. They took Ronald in and I know they like me. Wonder if they'd keep me, too. I bet they would.

I bet anything Aunt Pearl would let me stay with Ronald if I really wanted to. That's it! I'm gettin' outta here. Right now. I can't stand this place anymore or her.

I'll show her. I'll leave.

And I'll never come back.

The Kid walked into the house, holding his back erect with great effort, and into his bedroom. Masking the pain from the fall.

This time tomorrow I'm gonna have a happy home, goddamit, I'll show her.

He grabbed the box with his Cloverine Salve and pulled out the two dollars and change he'd collected from sales so far.

After listening for the rhythmic creaking of grandmother's rocking chair on the front porch, making sure she wasn't close enough to grab him or use some other device to pull his ass in check, the Kid slipped out, as quietly as he could, opening and closing the screen door with no more than a soft scratching sound from the spring and stepping lightly and quietly over the loose boards on the back porch.

To the back of the backyard, up through Miz Bollus' garden through an opening in the fence and up the rise to the Grainger's house where he knocked on the front screen door.

"Yeah?" Miz Grainger called from the kitchen at the back of the house.

"Larry here?"

"Yeah!" Larry.

"I thought you's home fer the night." He looked a hair puzzled as he opened the screen door and stepped down into the dirt-paved front yard.

"I wuz."

"What happened?"

"Oh, I run the bicycle into the locust tree and grandmother started in on me again. Sed I couldn't ever ride a bike again. I don't know. It jes' got to me, you know?"

"Yeah."

"So I'm takin' off. Fuck 'em. You wanna go with me?"

"I don't know. Momma and them'd be pretty upset if they didn't know whur I wuz. Let's thank 'bout it for a little while."

"I really hate to do it by myself, but I jes' can't live there no more, Larry. All she does is tell me everything I do is wrong and that I'm no account and that I'll always be no account. I can't take it anymore. You understand?"

"Hell yeah! You know I do. I couldn't live with that old woman fer a day. Hell yeah, I know what yer talking 'bout. Where you figger on goin?"

"I thought to my little brother's down between here and Puryear. Ain't too far. I don't think they'll think to catch me there."

"Well, okay, I guess I could go along. 'Course you understand, donchee, that I ain't going to stay, I'm jes' going along for the trip. You got any money?"

"Two dollars and change I took from my Cloverine Salve money."

"I ain't got no money but I can steal a couple packs of momma's Pall Malls from top of the frigerator. That should get us through a coupla days won't it?"

"Yeah."

"I'd really like to tell momma what we're doin', though. I hate fer her to worry like she's gonna do if she can't find me anywhere. You know momma, I'm pretty sure she won't tell nobody."

"But you don't know. We can't be sure. And I don't want grandmother to find out where I am."

"Yeah. Okay."

And so they sneaked away.

They kept to the underbrush, the back roads and the railroad.

A mile and a little more from home the Kid's back was already resonating with that deep pain he got when he stayed up too long or got tired or worried too much.

I gotta make it. I ain't going to go back. I don't wanna go back. I don't care how much it hurts my back. Ain't going to go back there. I don't have to stay with her and take that stuff. Gettin' to Ronald's will make all this worth it. And more!

The Old Paris and Murray Highway split off from U.S. 641 on the north side of town. Once they branched off the traffic lightened up and they could spend more of their energy on walking than on evading detection.

As the darkness intensified, so did the chill. The Kid was whipsawed between the sweat he worked up while he was walking — it didn't take long for him to become wringing wet from the exertion — and the chill of that sweat growing cold on his skin and in his shirt and pants. He was either burning up or freezing all night long.

"You really think this is a good idea, Kid?"

"I don't know, Larry. All I know is that I had to do somethin'."

The gravel road got long and rough the farther the unlikely duo crept along, its light-colored gravel forming a softly glowing path to the Kid's destiny. After three or four hours though, the Kid's rage subsided, leaving him wondering why the hell he'd ever thought this was going to work in the first place.

It ain't never goin' work. Aunt Pearl ain't goin' let me stay with Ronald and them. Grandmother ain't goin' let me stay there.

But, by God, I'll show 'em for a little while. I'll make grandmother sorry she ever treated me that way. Naw, she ain't ever been sorry before and she prob'ly not goin' start now.

Don't matter, though. None of this matters a bit right now because we're in the middle of the road in the middle of the night halfway out there and the only thing to do is finish this trip. God, am I tired!

When the Kid wasn't worrying or feeling sorry for himself the trip was indeed an adventure. From the smell of the night air which bespoke of mystery and wonder, to the looming, changing shapes of trees and bushes and weeds along the roadside — one minute offering themselves as friendly cover against attacking headlights — the next menacing the runaways with fierce shadow figures of destruction, on more than one occasion forcing the two to jump back out of harm's way.

Walk until he couldn't move, Larry the steadfast friend at his side. Then find a place out of sight of the road to sit and rest and smoke a cigarette, and even to catch a nap to ease his exhaustion in spite of the chill in the air.

Dragging themselves up and onward.

Finally the cutoff to Ronald's.

They made it the quarter mile or so down the road to Ronald's house without pause, pushed by the grace of a long downhill grade the very last part of the way.

"This is it. That's Ronald's house. We made it! I tell ya' man I had some doubts there for awhile. I didn't know whuther I could make it or not. The last two or three times we rested, it didn't feel like I could even git up again. And you ain't even tired."

"Oh yeah, don't you believe that. I'm plenty tired. I ain't ever walked this far at one time before. Bet it's ten miles or more we walked."

The pair walked through Ronald's front yard into the barnlot, into the barn and climbed onto the loft where they laid down behind some bales of hay, sure that they were too cold and too scared — though neither would admit that to the other — and too tired to sleep.

A rustling sound awoke the Kid. Startled, he sat up and listened. There it was again. With his fingers to his lips, the Kid told Larry to be quiet. He crawled over to the loft opening, peered down and saw his baby brother walking to and fro tending to his morning chores — rousting out six sleepy cows for their morning feed and milking before he took off for Puryear School.

"Hey!" the Kid called down.

You'da thought Ronald had been shot. He jumped 'bout six inches off the hard dirt floor of the barn and whirled around looking for the source of that voice.

"Watcha up to?" The Kid asked.

About then Ronald saw him peering over the edge of the loft opening.

"What the hell are you doin' here? You jes' about scared me to death."

"Sorry about that, Larry Grainger and me done run away from home."

"How'd you get here?"

"We walked."

275

"That's eight miles! You mean you walked the whole way?"

"Yep. We did. I couldn't think of anyplace else to go so we came here and came to the barn so we wouldn't disturb you durin' the night."

"What happened? What made you two want to run away anyhow?"

The Kid told Ronald the whole sordid story about how he'd been so sadly abused by grandmother and her never-ending stream of anti-Kid invective that he just had to leave.

"Well, you might as well come down from up there. Gotta tell Aunt Pearl and Uncle Ralph sooner or later. May's well be now I s'pose. Come on." And with a little snort he turned on his heels and started leading the way back to the house, the two recalcitrants bringing up the rear.

Somewhat to his surprise, the Kid saw his life and adventurous caper differently in sunlight than under the moon.

The chill had moved inward, he found, uncovering a shitload of doubts about whether this thing was going to work out at all and a dread of what was going to happen once they got to the big white house in a couple of minutes.

"Aunt Pearl! Uncle Ralph! Look here. See what the dog drug in!" Ronald called as he opened the kitchen's screen door.

Uncle Ralph, who was in the midst of starting a fire in the wood cookstove, glanced over, paused, and raised his bushy white eyebrows. "Well. Well. What have we got here? Where'd you fellows come from? You run-aways? How'd you get here? I don't suppose anybody knows where you are?"

Ronald briefed him and Aunt Pearl, who, by this time, was out of her rocking chair in the living room and standing in front of the boys with her eyes open wide and her face lighted up with a welcoming grin.

"Well, you might as well come in. I'll call Nellie and see if she'll get word to Larry's momma. Sit down there at the table and we'll have breakfast after awhile and figure this whole thing out."

Returning from her call to grandmother, Aunt Pearl's grin was even wider and more gleeful. "You kids stirred up quite a mess, I guess. Nellie says she and Miz Grainger have had the cops out searching for you all night. Said they've been looking everywhere, afraid y'all been hit by a car or something. And, for the first time since I know'd her, Nellie seemed like she was really worried about ye, Kid. Ain't that somethin'?"

While Ronald finished his chores, Aunt Pearl cooked up gravy and eggs and sausage and biscuits for everybody while Uncle Ralph sat and chuckled at the shenanigans.

The Kid would've rather walked into a buzzsaw than go back to grandmother's house, the last place in the world he wanted to live. But what could he do?

Aunt Pearl and Uncle Ralph haven't said a word about I could live here. It could have been, he thought, because they were poor and simply couldn't afford it.

I can't live at Aunt Louise's and Uncle Nolan's. They had a houseful.

The Watson's were dirt farmers barely scratching out a living.

There ain't no place I can go except back there. I guess I'll jes' lie and act like I'm real sorry, like this was a bad mistake or something.

At least I've got Larry to play with unless Miz Grainger puts a stop to that because of last night; she'll prob'ly think I'm a bad influence on him and not want me to mess around with him anymore.

I wish Aunt Pearl and Uncle Ralph would let me live here with them and Ronald. Don't they know why I ran away? Shit!

Larry talked to his mom who was at grandmother's house and started blubbering about how he was sorry and he didn't know what he was doing and he didn't know it was going to hurt anybody and he was awfully, awfully sorry.

Booohooo. Booofuckinghooo.

The Kid talked to grandmother. Rather, grandmother talked at the Kid. "Kid, if you come back here, you gotta promise you'll do better. Kid, I don't wanchee here if yer goin' keep on pullin' this kind of trick. Hear me?"

"Yes ma'am."

"Are you sure ye wanna come back?"

"Yes ma'am."

"Will you promise to straighten up and do better and show me some respect?"

"Yes ma'am."

"Okay, you c'n come on home then."

278

Larry and the Kid sat in the living room with long faces, looking out the window until they finally heard the crunching of a car coming down the hill. The Kid and Larry walked onto the porch to await Larry's sentencing. The Kid would have to wait a little longer for his.

At least until he got back to grandmother's house.

To the Kid's surprise, Miz Grainger said hardly anything. "Boy, ye shore gave us a fit of worryin' last night. What in the world got into ye? Walkin' all this way?" She looked at Aunt Pearl. "Thank ye for feedin' 'em and holdin' on to 'em whilst I could come down and pick 'em up. Miz Sutton says to say thanks, too."

The trip back was made mostly in silence. The Kid was so nervous the heel of his right foot kept tapping like he was keeping time with music. He'd've rather died than face grandmother's verbal firing squad.

The Kid got out of the car, climbed the steps, walked past grandmother and went directly to his room where he sat still and quietly as he tried to make himself disappear from the face of the earth.

Grandmother entered the house. He could hear her walk through the living room and the kitchen toward him.

"What in the world did ye think you's doin', Kid? I declare I don't know what I'm goin' to do with ye. I can't do no more. I can't. Now ye tol' me on the phone that you're goin' to straighten up and fly right, didn't ye?"

"Yes ma'am."

"Well, I'm gonna take ye at yer word cause I haf to. I ain't got no choice, do I?"

"No, ma'am."

"Git yerself ready fer school."

I can't stand it, this being fussed at. Haven't ye gotta do somethin' when you feel like you can't take anymore?

I can't take anymore of your fussin' so I ran away. I'd never a' run away if I'd known I was gonna have to come back and face y'all.

I'm bad. I'm bad. I'm bad! Are ye happy with that? I fucked up. Is that what you want to hear?

I really didn't mean to hurt anybody; all I wanted to do was get away from here, away from you and go somewhere where I could ride a bicycle and have fun without somebody always trying to mess it up. That's all I wuz doin.

If I Could Only Whistle

John Frank Marcum was born in Tennessee in eighteen-eighty-five. He went to work for the railroad when he was a young man, working his way up to engineer of steam engines and then to diesels for the last few years before he retired from the Louisville and Nashville line which most everybody called the L & N.

Mister Marcum was in his early seventies by the time the Kid and he became friends. A couple years previously the cardiovascular boogeyman had zapped Mister Marcum's ass near 'bouts into the grave.

The Kid could remember that before his retirement Mister Marcum would take off before the good light of day and not return until two or three days later. Those trips were perfect fodder for the rich imaginations of kids like the Kid and Larry Grainger in whose fantasies railroading was right up there next to chasing bad guys on the topside of Trigger and Champion.

The Kid was one of the few kids in a non-railroad family in Rorie Addition who had actually ridden on a train, thanks to the evil viri.

Railroad heroes were scattered throughout the neighborhood. Mister Flynn used to give the Kid expired union pins that he would wear on one of the railroad man's secondhand caps. Mister Grainger — Larry's father, Dalton — was a fireman. The guy who, until the early fifties, stoked coal into the furnaces that drove the steam engines. Mister Marcum had the best job of them all. He was the engineer. That meant he drove the train.

The first time the Kid saw the inside of the Marcum house was when Miz Marcum had agreed to chaperone him to Memphis for a post-polio checkup. Later grandmother and he would go down there by special invitation to watch the television on a Friday or Saturday night.

The Kid hadn't had a lot of male role models he was wont to take after, and Mister Marcum was a warm comfort station along that route. They were good times, the times when the Kid could fantasize Mister Marcum was his father.

The very best moments in the Kid's life with Mister Marcum had to do with fishing. That old man taught the Kid the joys of chasing underwater food with a hook and a worm or doughball. Going fishing with Mister Marcum was one of the precious few grandmother approved Kid activities.

Mister Marcum mostly provided himself with his own fishing supplies. Worms from his very own worm farm, which consisted of a number three wash tub he'd sunk in his backyard and seeded with a few of those big earthworms. The only thing he ever had to pay for when they went on one of their fishing trips was gasoline.

The TVA was created in an attempt to improve the steadily worsening conditions in the Tennessee River Basin which suffered from frequent and destructive floods, intermittent navigability of the river, deforestation, and severely eroded land. The Springville pump house was a part of all that flood control.

It was to the backwaters of the Springville levee and pump house that Mister Marcum and the Kid rushed off to whenever Mister Marcum got a hankering to dip a hook or two. It was also where the Kid learned everything he would ever need to know about fishing.

It would be just about breaking daylight when they pulled onto the hillside running down to the pump house and parked the car. They'd load themselves down with rods, reels, fishnet, tackle box, a sackful of sardines and crackers, and empty burlap bags for hauling their catch home that night.

Then they'd walk down to the pump house and up a well-beaten path alongside the backwaters until the Kid thought he was going to drop. Finally Mister Marcum would see something that would satisfy him and stop to make their base camp.

A half dozen poles were set. Then it was the Kid's turn. He got an open reel and rod, one that would be real hard to fuck up. "Here, you take this rod. Bait it with the redworms and cast it up and down the bank here where ye see some brush or grass stickin' outta the water. That's where the bream beds are like to be."

There was no bigger thrill for the Kid than that instant when he knew for sure he'd hooked a fish. It was as if the fish, in pulling the line in his effort to escape, was pulling a ripcord that flooded the Kid with adrenaline for the ensuing battle. What a rush. Face flushing. Hands and arms moving furiously for half a second to make doubly sure it was true and to set the hook in the fish's mouth or throat or belly.

The smallest panfish fought like a behemothic monster when it was struggling for its life. The Kid never quite figured out how he could hook a ten pound fish, nearly break his line reeling it in, and yet somehow end up with a little shirttail of a thing when it broke the surface of the water. Every damn time.

And so the Kid walked up and down a half mile or so of the creek bank, throwing his wormed hook into the water every fifteen feet or so, and, if it didn't bite in five or ten minutes, he'd reel it in and go on over to the next hope.

Mister Marcum's and his paths would cross once in awhile.

They did not chitchat while they fished. Fishing was a serious business. Mister Marcum said it was and the Kid believed him, and behaved like someone who believed him and wanted to do it again sometime. Because he sorely did.

Every once in awhile the Kid would see one of the sapling poles bending over with its nose under water, the signal that a doughball had been sucked down. He'd grab the pole and pull the fish out of the water and throw it into a toesack. [That's what knowledgeable folks called burlap bags.] He'd tie the toesack to a tree on the bank and toss the fish and the sack back into the water. That way the fish got protection from the prying jaws of hungry other fishes and stayed alive and fresh enough to get eaten by hungry people when they got home.

"Y'ready to eat a little somethin' for lunch, boy?"

"Yessir."

"Y'like sardines, boy?"

"Yessir." The first time Mister Marcum asked him that, the Kid didn't have the slightest idea what sardines tasted like; still he responded with his patented, "Yessir." Ten minutes later Mister Marcum's end-of-lunch signal sounded.

Infrequently, Miz Marcum would accompany the two guys. The Kid liked that, too. She made the day go more quickly. She talked and always brought little snacks and goodies they could share while Mister Marcum was doing the serious stuff up the creek a ways.

After lunchtime, the afternoon was a reprise of the morning. The afternoon was the Kid's favorite part. He got tired about four o'clock and he'd find himself a tree to sit down and lean against, and became more interested in life around him, especially the afternoon sun which soothed him with its lazy rays.

Thence the long-ass walk back to the car parked on the hillside. The more fish they had caught, the heavier their load and the longer the trip seemed. Once the gear was stowed in the trunk the Kid had the treat of his day, sitting down in the car, so damned comfortable after the long day the Kid would have purred if he could have.

Mister Marcum died on the day of the Kid's twenty-fourth birthday.

A Christmas Present

Uncle Ralph pulled the car off U.S. 69, just south of the Paris city limits, and into Eakers parking lot, stopping just short of the gas pumps. The concrete block main building was set off the road thirty or forty feet and was almost hidden behind ice machines, minnow tanks, and the like.

Aunt Pearl turned her head around from the front seat. "I'll go get him and bring him out to the car. Ain't no need of you having to go in there." She opened the car door and heaved herself out into the night and on into Eakers Store.

Eakers was a sportsman store and grill. It opened up at three o'clock in the morning for hunters and fishermen to stop in for breakfast, bait, bullets, gasoline and whatever else they needed for their blood quests. Business slowed down during the day to folks who'd come by for breakfast or to shoot the shit with whoever was manning the store.

At night – *Shazam!* – Eakers magically transformed itself into a real southern country beer joint. Early in the evening people would come by to eat fried catfish and hushpuppies and drink a beer or two. By the time supper was over, the dozen tables and booths would start filling with regulars who came to palaver and drink beer. Talk a lot. Drink a lot. Beat a path to the outdoor toilets on the south side of the place.

The Kid had never been inside of Eakers. Mister and Miz Marcum had stopped here with him in the car two or three times but they always brought the beer and cold drinks out to the car where he waited.

Uncle Ralph and Ronald were taciturn. The Kid was scared to death at the prospect of reuniting with his father, the man grandmother, Uncle Jay and others had been painting as a monster. "No tellin' what Connie Moody'd do if y'all wust to go back there. It's a wonder he ain't come and stole ye jest for the meanness uv it." He wondered that he wasn't shaking as bad on the outside as he was on the inside where a mixer was running wild through his guts.

In what must've been no more than a few moments, the Kid turned his head at the sound of a door closing and approaching footsteps crunching gravel quietly. Holding his breath as he saw Aunt Pearl come out, leading a man with a strangely familiar face and walk, who kinda shuffled along like a shy schoolboy.

He was not a tall man. He was not a handsome man but it seemed like to the Kid that he was a powerful man. When he lifted his half bald head and met the Kid's eyes, the Kid saw, and felt, that familiar circuit which had energized him so many years ago – had connected him to a father and family that had been all but reduced to faint memories of something that resembled contentment.

But still his head reeled from fright as all of grandmother's ominous warnings raced up and down and around his nervous system, spinning his mind round and round and round until he felt like he was going to fall and puke his guts out from the dizziness.

Aunt Pearl brought him over to the side of the car where the Kid was sitting with the window down. "Know who this is?" She asked the Kid.

No response.

"Well, this is yer daddy, Kid."

"Hi."

The second thing that hit the Kid with a slap was that Connie Taylor Moody didn't look anything like the monster grandmother had painted him over the years. Nor was he acting like a monster. And it didn't look like he was drunk, either.

"Hey."

And so it was thusly that the Kid was reunited with his father, for the first time since Jacky and he had walked away from that locked up old log house hand in hand some nine years earlier.

"How ya doin'?"

"Okay."

"I'm real glad to see ye."

No response.

"Pearl says you're doin' right smartly in school."

"Yes sir."

This was not the first time Ronald had seen dad. Aunt Pearl had arranged for several previous meetings. She said it was because the kids should know who their father was, no matter who he was.

She had decided that the appropriate time for the Kid to meet dad was Christmas time. And so it had been. This was a week or so after Christmas in fifty-eight.

No hug.

No handshake.

Nothing like that entered the Kid's mind.

He didn't know whether dad thought about it and didn't or didn't think about it and didn't.

After allowing what she considered to be adequate time for a family reunion, Aunt Pearl shoved past dad to hand the Kid a gift-wrapped box. "Here's a Christmas present from your daddy."

The Kid took it, drew it into the car and sat there looking at it.

Not moving.

"Go 'head. Open it." Aunt Pearl.

"Okay," as he tore at the paper and box to find a plaid short-sleeved shirt with button-down collar. There were blues and blacks in the shirt. The Kid didn't particularly like plaid.

Mixed feelings, most of which he couldn't begin to articulate. One which he could was, "Thank you." And he meant it. Tears halfway up to his eyes.

"Is that the right size? I's just goin' on what Pearl sed 'bout how big you are."

"It looks like it."

Nobody said Dad. Nobody said Son.

"And here's yours, Ronald." Aunt Pearl shoved another package past dad and the Kid.

Another shirt.

"Thanks." Ronald was a mirror of his dad in some of his facial and vocal expressions way back then. That kind of half grin and the way he'd swing his head around half way to emphasize that he's talking to you.

The rest of that first visit was wrapped in a fog that filled the Kid's mind.

That it had come about at all is a tribute to Aunt Pearl. A reunion of people who had once been so close was not a bad thing. Less than a decade previously the Kid and Jacky and dad and Annie Catherine had been as tight as any group of four people could be.

Cooking slumgullion in a pot over the fireplace while dad took down the guitar and sang bawdy songs with Catherine's voice chiming in, a bell in perfect pitch.

Going everywhere together: to bars, barbecues, drunken bacchanalias, on food gathering forays to steal chickens and corn and watermelons from black folks who wouldn't tell even if they caught them 'cause they were white.

At first only Ronald and the Kid were in contact with dad. Within a short period of time, Jacky started visiting him and, eventually, Peggy and Joe Frankie stopped by Eaker's to say hi, too.

The Kid would eventually wind up closest to dad, perhaps because he had that black hole of need that near swallowed up his soul and which could be fed only by dad, a theory that turned out to be mostly true. After dad's death the hole was left with its maws open forevermore.

After Jacky and the Kid left, dad and Annie Catherine remained married for eight more years. Although marriage almost certainly didn't accurately describe the nature of their relationship. They stayed together, off and on. Frequenting Henry County's beer joints. Gettin' drunk and fighting. Making up.

From all accounts theirs was not a monogamous relationship. There were rumors of whoring and pimping and such. Dad never denied them when in later years he would talk about his life with the Kid.

One thing that was obvious is that both their lives ran out of control for years. The Kid would take some small measure of comfort in the fact that his father hadn't had to spiral downward in search of that unfindable peace all by hisself, even if only for a short spell.

Dad never learned to return to real life after mom died. Annie Catherine was just a young mother when dad hooked up with her and she certainly did seem to enjoy the "good life", the glamour she found inside the can of Country Club and inside the bottle of peach brandy, mixed liberally with like-minded minds and arm benders around town.

After the divorce dad became a sort of migrant worker. He worked some as a farm hand for Pete Valentine, then went down to Louisiana where he cooked on an oil rig, and finally back to Henry County where he spent the rest of his life moving from beer joint to beer joint, making a circuit for himself. He was on the move constantly exercising the hell out of a treadmill.

Dad was a mean drunk. He didn't give a shit about size or whether you were the law or a murdering horse thief, he'd jump your ass and do his best to chop it up and shove it down your throat. Or if he couldn't and you beat the piss out of him, so be it! What the fuck! He had a death wish. He had to have had. Otherwise he wouldn't have waded in on anybody for any reason. Or no reason at all. One of his opponents slashed dad's lower lip all the way through. But would he go to a doctor or a hospital to get it sewn up? Hell no. He let it heal itself if it wanted to and if it didn't he didn't give a damn. And it did heal, although his lower lip was forevermore out of line by a good quarter of an inch.

Dad did a whole lot of time in the Henry County Jail. The sheriff and his deputies got to know him well over the years. His habits. His temper. Inevitably, sooner or later they'd show up where he was picking a fight. "You want a piece of Connie Moody? Come on. You might git a piece, but Connie Moody don't give a shit and you'll know he wuz there. Come on! Connie Moody ain't takin' no shit from nobody, not even you. I don't kere how many guns and badges you got. Connie Moody'll shove 'em all up yer ass. I ain't skeered uv nobody. You hear me?"

The next morning Connie Moody would wake up in the Henry County Jail in Paris.

Again.

Covered with bruises.

Again.

Sore as hell from his eyeballs to his toenails. Proof of his enduring bravery in the face of the foe.

Again.

Times a thousand.

The same scenarios.

The same people.

Groundhog Day.

There was no stopping him or shushing him once he got a head of steam built. Offering him a ride home would just piss him off worse. Warn him he'd wind up arrested if he didn't calm down a little and he'd laugh in their faces.

Doctor Jekyll and Mister Hyde. Sober, dad was as affable and likeable a person as you could find anywhere. Even the people who found themselves arresting him time after time liked him.

When he wasn't drinking.

Hard working.

Friendly.

Give you the shirt off his back.

Cooperative.

When he wasn't drinking.

Momma! Momma! You shore took the starch outta that man by dyin' on him. Momma! Momma! Donchu know what you done? Lookit! Lookit!

Only thang in the world that man of yours looks forward to is dyin' too. Momma! Oohh! Momma! What you done did, woman. What you done did?

The Kid was thirty years old when dad died in Veterans Hospital in Nashville. By then the two of them had become good friends, had spent untold hours drinking beer and talking about their lives and everything else.

Dad said it wasn't true that he didn't try to come and get Jacky and me. Like he'd tried to go get Peggy and Ronald after they'd been taken away. "I tried, Kid, I don't know how many times I tried. Catherine and me would drive up there to your grandmother's to get ye and every time we went there wuz somebody wouldn't even let us outta the car. Wouldn't even let me see y'all, much less bring ye home with me. Don't ever thank I didn't try. I did. I ain't saying ye woulda had the best home in the world. You remember how bad it was at times before? Well, it didn't git any better. Matter of fact, it got a lot worse sometimes after y'all were gone."

"I can't tell ye some of the thangs I've done to keep alive. Thangs me and Catherine both done. A whole lot we ain't proud of. But don't never let nobody tell ye Connie Moody didn't try to come back and get y'all after ye went to liv with yer grandmother. Cause I was there seems like a hunnert times or more. I was there. They jes' never would let me in. Listen to me, Kid. I tried."

Perhaps.

Perhaps Connie Moody had to drink. To try and replenish all the tears he shed between nineteen-forty-seven and nineteen-seventy-three.

Perhaps.

The Kid did think a lot about the truth. Wondering about just what was and just what wasn't, and who told it and who didn't and just what the hell was it all about, anyhow.

There was no answer. From God. Or anybody else. Anywhere else.

Perhaps there are indeed extant multiple universes which are identical and simultaneous except for what we do in them.

Say, in one universe I grow up to be a monk, conscientious and god-fearing while in another I make normal satyrs jealous as hell with my rampaging sexual escapades. But what if there is a common consciousness among all those aspects in all those universes? What if, at some level, they all meet on Tuesday nights to play poker and discuss the week's events?

And then what if I occasionally wake up thinking I'm in universe A when in fact I'm in universe C but carry on as if I'm in universe A? That would explain all these apparent discrepancies, wouldn't it?

Yeah! That's the ticket.

...

In 1960 I was among a group of students led by our teacher, Miss Ruby, to a statewide speech contest in Nashville, TN. I was a newbie, and the competition was embarrassingly (to me) fierce.

"The men met together at last, the men who had played god…" I will never forget the opening words of my dissertation. I was so nervous I gave my competitors a copy of my lines and asked them to prompt me when I got stuck!

Afterwards I skipped out on the awards ceremony, choosing instead to opt for pizza with a couple of comely coeds from the host school. After impressing the ladies with my pubescent wit and charm, it was time to meet up with my fellow students and get on home.

I was fully prepared to engage in the requisite after-date puffery, but was wholly unprepared for the shining trophy which was waiting for me.

A foot high brass pronouncement of my superlative speech skills. State Champion. National Forensic League. I was a big fucking deal. Something nobody could, or did, ever take away, in title or in spirit. Fifty some odd years later and that tarnish-tinged cup is still readily, and comfortingly, within my sight.

...

...

Grandmother, for some reason unknown to me, refused to give me a key to our house. Always assuring me that she would awaken and answer my knocks should the need arise.

I climbed the stairs and walked the porch toward the door, with a lightness of step that must have come from the day's success.

I knocked.

No answer.

I knocked again. A dozen times.

No answer. Any of the times.

Now I'm thinking that grandmother's either dead or, at the very least, sick and unable to roust herself out of bed.

I walked around the house to her bedroom window and knocked. And knocked. And knocked.

To no avail.

Not a peep was to be heard from either my grandmother or her bed springs.

I walked to the neighbor's house down the hill and phoned Uncle Telous, who got in his car and fetched me to his and Aunt Maxine's house for the night. But not before he tried to wake up grandmother hisself.

The next morning, grandmother was all kinds of curious as to why I hadn't come home the night before. She didn't believe a word from us, not even from the sainted lips of trusted Uncle Telous.

No matter how fervent our protestations, I believe she went to her grave disbelieving that she could possibly have slept through all that clatter.

...

RAMBLINGS
by flee

When I was twenty-one:
    passing for physically normal
    my energy was young
    my effort enormous
    hid any semblance of being a cripple
    I liked being a reporter
    I adored my job
    I would fake it
    I walked a mile a day to build my energy
    I bought a weight set to build my muscles
    I welcomed John Barleycorn to mask my exhaustion
    I passed
    I hid the pain
    I hid the exhaustion
    I didn't
    I couldn't
    "Don't walk with your hand in your pocket."
    The hand was pushing the leg to make me walk
When I was twenty-five:
    an assignment reporter
    much walking
    from where I parked to the city-county building
    from the parking lot to the press conference
    from the car to the murder scene
    half a dozen times a day
    the exhaustion grows
    I must mask it
    I can't let them know
    does everybody get this tired?
    thank god they're pushing me up to that
        welfare mother's apartment
    could I have made it without them?

Wallace, Humphrey and Nixon, rushing
        after them
And the Tigers, the new world champs
I can't let them see
I must not let them know
I know what they'll do
I've seen them do it
But what can I do?
I'm so...so tired
[unfinished]

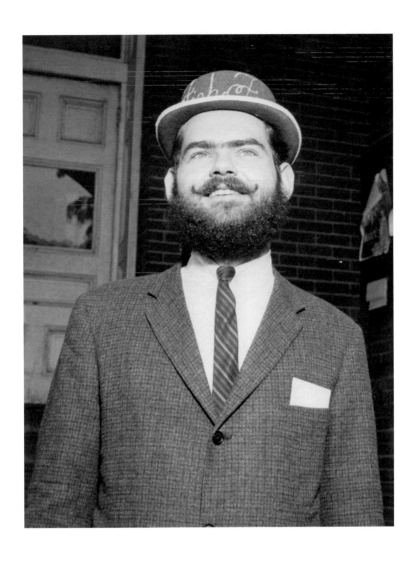

Frankie Lee Moody
King of the Catfish Whisker Contest
Winner ~ **"Most Magnificent Beard"**
Age 20
Paris, Tennessee ~ 1963

80 for the 80s

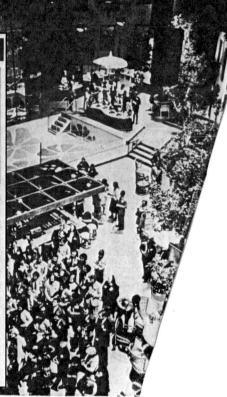

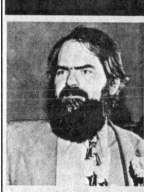

Frank Lee, 36, Broadview Heights, public affairs director for radio stations WHK-AM and WMMS-FM. One of the creative minds that has shaped programming on two of Cleveland's most listened-to stations, Lee calls his job "one of the most insane yet devised by the demented mind of man."

Second strike
State Journal 4-11-87

Polio survivor fights a resurgence of the disease

By JAMES A. HARRIS
Lansing State Journal

When he began falling down in public places a few years ago, Frank Lee was perplexed.

Lee, 43, of Lansing, a survivor of a childhood bout with polio, thought he had left that portion of his life behind forever. He never considered his disease as a cause for his falls.

But, like many polio survivors, Lee is finding he must face the onslaught of a second strike from the dreaded disease.

He was among about 200 polio survivors gathering in Lansing Saturday for the second annual meeting at the Plymouth Congregational Church of Michigan's POLIO NETWORK.

The 900-member strong organization formed to help survivors cope with the changes in their later years.

"After junior high school I was basically able to pass for normal — that is there was no outward sign I was handicapped — and get into broadcasting," said Lee, who is married and the father of an 11-year-old daughter.

He said he worked in radio and television broadcasting in several states when he suddenly began collapsing in 1978 while working in Cleveland. "I would just fall in a heap," said Lee. "Then it started

to get so I wouldn't be able to get up by myself.

"I don't know if you've ever experienced anything like that, but I can tell you it was terribly embarrassing," he said.

He attributed the episodes to a lack of exercise. Later, when exhaustion set in he decided to take a break from work. He then heard the late effects of polio and its symptoms being discussed.

"It was like someone was discussing some of the things that were happening to me," he said.

Now, he said, he can only walk short distances with crutches, depending mostly on a motorized chair. He lives off Social Security disability compensation.

The resurgence of the disease in his body has taken its toll psychologically, he said. He now works on telling other potential victims what is happening to their bodies.

"I didn't know for four years what was happening to me," Lee said.

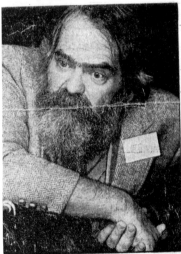

Lansing State Journal/GREG DeRUITER

Frank Lee of Lansing survived childhood bout with polio.

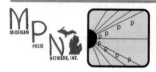

POLIO
PERSPECTIVES

VOL 27 NO 3 FALL 2012

Promoting Understanding Though the Michigan Polio Network, Inc Since 1986

FRANK LEE, FOUNDER & FIRST EDITOR OF THE
POLIO PERSPECTIVES NEWSLETTER & MPN LEGEND

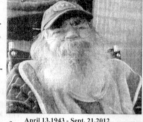

April 13,1943 - Sept. 21,2012

Frank Lee passed away on September 21, 2012 with cherished friend, Connie Breitbeil, by his side. Frank leaves behind daughter Connie, granddaughter Gabrielle and grandson Jacob in Michigan as well as brothers, sisters and extended family in Kentucky & Tennessee. He happily left his c-pap, oxygen tanks, wardrobe of wheelchairs, and an army of pillows. Frank came to the First Statewide Post Polio Conference in 1985 at the invitation of Charlene Bozarth. Back then, he alternated between crutches and a wheelchair. On his blog, frankieleeee.wordpress.com, Frank speaks of his severe depression when his ability to maintain a successful career as a journalist disappeared as his body failed him. " I thought all hope of any hope for my life was gone. A career down the tubes... A body quickly following suit... But Janice and Charlene, then-president of MPN, pumped and punched and pounded and pled until I started breathing again. Very Slowly at first..." "We need a newsletter, boy; can you put one together for us?" Yes, he did. We needed a journalist; God sent us our own Hemingway. We have reaped the benefits ever since. Thank you, Frank Lee with all our hearts. (*more of Frank on page 2*)